HITCH FIT Living
Cookbook

100+ Recipes for your fit life!

Diana Chaloux LaCerte

&

Micah LaCerte

Important Copyright Infringement Warning:
Please be aware that Federal copyright law protects all information provided to you
in your Hitch Fit Living Cookbook. It is illegal to re-sell, re-send, copy, auction, share,
or give away this program. Violators will be prosecuted in a court of law. Thank you
in advance for your compliance.

Your Hitch Fit Living Cookbook is not intended as medical counseling or medical
advice. The information contained herein should not be used to treat, diagnose or
prevent a disease or medical condition without the advice of a medical professional.

CONTENTS

INTRODUCTION

Hitch Fit is the number one Online Personal Training System in the world, promoting healthy living and weight loss via proper training and nutrition. Hitch Fit is not about quick fixes, but true lifestyle transformation. Founded by top personal trainers, "transformers", and world champion fitness models Micah LaCerte & Diana Chaloux - Lacerte. Hitch Fit is based in Kansas City, MO where they own and operate 2 personal training facilities. This cookbook features healthy Hitch Fit lifestyle recipes. If you are interested in Hitch Fit's transformation programs, visit www.hitchfit.com.

ACKNOWLEDGMENTS

Thanks to all of our clients worldwide who have committed to the Hitch Fit lifestyle and our motto to Believe – Transform – Inspire. You all are OUR inspiration to continue striving to make this world a healthier place! Thank you to Linda Mosse for all her cooking expertise and editing skills in helping us bring this book to life.

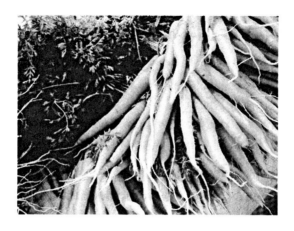

CHAPTER 1

TRANSFORMING YOUR THOUGHTS ON FOOD

Hitch Fit is a lifestyle. It is about changing your mind, your body and ultimately your life and fulfilling your true potential throughout your journey here on earth! Many of you are reading this cookbook because you have already joined us at Hitch Fit and are progressing into a maintenance phase. These recipes will aid you in continuing in your successful journey to maintain your transformation. If you have not yet begun, or have not yet reached out to us, please don't hesitate to contact as at www.HitchFit.com so we can help you get started on your journey to wellness. If this is your first time hearing about Hitch Fit, then we would like to extend a big hello and welcome to you! Whether you picked up this cookbook for new ideas for your "already fit" lifestyle, or you are just embarking on a journey towards improved health, we are delighted to be a part of your fitness journey. We encourage you to get directly connected with us via our websites and social media. All of our links will be provided for you at the back of this book, and we would love you to join our positive community and get to know us better!

In our first book, Hitch Fit: Keys to Transforming Your Life, we concentrated on why it is crucial to have a transformation regarding your thoughts and actions in relation to exercise and nutrition. Our motto is Believe – Transform – Inspire. You first have to believe that you are capable of succeeding, understand that you have the power and responsibility to change your life, and then implement the tools and strategies to get your physique exactly where you want it to be! We've seen thousands of clients worldwide go through incredible transformations when they really embraced healthy eating and exercise as a way of life. Their stories are amazing and powerful and we hope that you stop by the Hitch Fit site to check them out.

When our clients go through the "transformation" phase, we believe in keeping things simple when it comes to nutrition. That means sticking with the basics and really getting to know your foods by reading labels, measuring portions and learning WHAT you need to eat and WHEN you need to eat it. During transformation we don't encourage the use of a lot of fancy recipes just because it can get confusing, and portion control can be more difficult. We've found, after working with thousands of clients, that keeping food choices simple and easy during transformation is what will get you most efficiently to your goals.

Throughout the pages of this, our first ever healthy recipes book, you will find SOME recipes that would coincide with what we approve of for transformation periods. However, the majority of these recipes are going to be best for once you have gone through transformation and are in a place where your goal is to maintain your fit and healthy physique. These recipes are also great for anyone who is not mentally and emotionally prepared to commit to total transformation, but do want to start making some smart and easy changes to their eating habits. Even by making smarter food choices, you can make great improvements to your health by losing weight through the incorporation of more whole foods and by eliminating the junk food from your diet.

In this Hitch Fit Living Cookbook, we want to go into more detail on some wonderful recipes and food options that will fit right in with your fit and healthy lifestyle.

On average, we say this to people 2 to 3 times per day: "Abs are NOT made in the gym. They are made in the kitchen." This statement is absolutely true and pertains not just to being able to see a "six pack" set of abs but also to any other physical fitness goal that you might have such as leaner legs, glutes, arms, hips, etc. The desire to have any one of these is only doable if you are willing to spend some time in the kitchen as well as the gym. When our clients go through transformation, many of them get those visual abs or leaner physiques that they are going for, but once you are there, the ONLY way to maintain it is also through your choices in the kitchen! This recipe book will give you some great ideas on delicious foods to eat to keep that fit body for the rest of your life.

Hitch Fit is very education-focused. We don't want you to eat certain foods just because we said so. We want you to know WHY you are eating them and what they are going to do for you. There is no single diet plan that works for EVERY body. Figuring out how to lose weight is a matter of figuring out YOUR body. Losing weight, shedding body fat and maintaining a fit physique for life boils down to understanding some key pieces of information regarding food. Each of the recipes in your book includes nutritional information on items such as calories, protein, fats, carbohydrates and sugar. It's important for you to know what these terms mean and how each of these things affects your body, so we will go over this in more detail now.

Calorie Consumption and Metabolism

First, it is helpful to understand calorie consumption versus calorie expenditure. A calorie is simply a unit of energy. If you are consuming more energy than your body is utilizing to function in a day, then that energy has to be stored somewhere. If it isn't used right away, it can either be stored in muscles as glycogen to be used at a later time for energy, or it stores as fat. The bottom line is that in order to lose weight and shed body fat, you have to be consuming less than you are expending in a day. When you are maintain weight, that means that you are consuming about the same amount of calories per day that you are expending, and in a situation where you are trying to gain muscle mass, that would mean you were eating in surplus of the calories you were expending.

It seems like weight loss or maintenance or muscle gain would be easy right? Well, not really. If it were JUST about calories in versus calories out, then a lot of the bad habits we have might actually work. Starvation diets would be an effective way to get lean, or you could just eat Twinkies all day and get lean, or you could not eat in the morning and then eat all your caloric intake for the day in the evening, and still get lean. Or in order to maintain your weight you could just eat a giant serving of your maintenance calories at one sitting and not gain anything! We hear over and over again from people with these types of habits. They don't understand why they are still GAINING weight, even when they are not eating above their calorie recommendations for the day.

Here's the thing. Your body is smart, and it can only utilize a certain amount of fuel at a time. Overloading your system with a massive calorie consumption in one sitting is like trying to pour 20 gallons of fuel into a 10 gallon tank, and then wondering why it's all spilling out. Your body also can tell when it is starving. When you go for long periods of time without eating, you are sending signals to your body that you will not be feeding it for quite some time. Your body will respond by sending an alert to all systems to SLOW down and preserve as much energy as possible. It also encourages your body to store fat because during this time of famine, the most important thing is that your body survives!

Your metabolism, the rate at which your body burns off calories in order to sustain itself, is slowed down significantly when you are starving yourself and are not getting a sufficient amount of calories to perform daily functions. That makes it even slower at processing food as energy. This, in turn, contributes to the vicious cycle of fat gain, even IF your calorie consumption isn't over what your daily caloric intake should be.

***The lesson to learn here is that you DO have to be in a calorie deficit in order to lose body fat. If you consume over what you are expending in a day, it will store as fat. This overspill simply has no place else to go! But the other rule to remember is that your body can only utilize a small amount of calories at a time, so eating all your calories at once or starving your body throughout the day and only eating 1 or 2 times daily, will be counterproductive to shedding body fat and getting lean!

During maintenance phases, your calories can and will be higher than when you are losing fat weight, but you DO still have to be aware of the foods that you are eating, when you are eating them and how much of them you are eating! What often happens is people go on a "diet" for a period of time, then as soon as they have lost all the scale weight (not necessarily body fat) that they wanted, they go right back to eating what they were before, and then scratch their heads wondering why they didn't maintain their weight loss! This is the key reason why healthy eating is such a critical part of maintaining your fit and healthy lifestyle. Making healthy choices for the rest of your life is worth it, it's an amazing way to eat and to live!

Types of Calories

The type of calories you are consuming is just as important as the amount of calories you eat. There are foods that will promote fat gain regardless of if you go over your caloric needs (i.e. high sugar and high fat foods). If you think that fat loss or weight maintenance is as simple as a matter of calories in versus calories out, then you ought to be able to eat candy, cookies and Twinkies all day as long as you are eating fewer calories than your body is expending. Wouldn't that make sense and be true? Let's take a closer look.

FOOD CLASSIFICATION

Foods are classified into different categories: protein, carbohydrates, and fats. They are all essential to your diet and to your overall health. Let's take a look at these categories in a bit more depth. They include protein, carbohydrates and fats, and eating them in the proper combinations will aid you in transforming your body into the fit physique you desire and maintaining it for life.

PROTEIN

What is protein, and why do our bodies need it? Protein is the main building block for your fit and healthy body. There are a lot of great benefits to eating protein. We already know that it aids in muscle building, repairs body tissue and preserves lean muscle tissue. Protein also aids in immune function and aids in body fat loss as it stimulates the metabolism. Protein will keep you feeling full and will help you to overcome any cravings to make unhealthy food choices.

Protein is made up of amino acids, which are essential to the human body. They aid in the development of muscle and muscle growth and repair. They are responsible for all of the body's enzymes and also play a key role in sleep, normalizing moods, concentration and attention. When you eat protein, your stomach and small intestines break it down into amino acids, which can then be utilized for all of these functions. If you don't consume enough protein, your body will not be able to build or maintain lean muscle mass. In fact, you will actually lose precious muscle tissue because your body will have to use it for fuel. The reason you don't want this to happen is because your metabolism will slow down and your body will not be as efficient at burning fat.

In order to achieve a lean physique, your body must be burning fat and not muscle. To ensure that you consume enough protein, a good rule of thumb is to ingest 1 to 2 grams of protein per pound of body weight per day. If you are looking to maintain the muscle you currently have and burn off fat, you will want to stick to about 1 gram per pound. If your goal is to gain additional muscle mass you will want to increase that amount and consume around 1.5 to 2 grams per pound of bodyweight. There is no need to eat more than the recommended amounts of protein. If you consume more than your body can utilize, it will go to waste and will be excreted.

Protein is also a very thermic food, meaning that it takes a lot of energy to break it down in digestion. This means that more calories are burned when you eat protein than any other type of food. Up to 20% of calories consumed from a protein source can potentially be burned up in the digestion process, just another reason why it is such an important staple of nutrition and maintaining a fit healthy physique.

There are two types of proteins: complete and incomplete. Complete proteins are found in most products of animal origin, such as meat, poultry, eggs, cheese, fish and milk. They are called "complete" because they contain all of the amino acids that are essential to your body.

Complete proteins should be consumed at every single meal, some protein sources have a higher biological value than others, meaning that they are more readily used by your body as far as muscle repair and retention goes. Animal proteins have a higher biological value than vegetable proteins for example. But that being said

Here is a list of food sources that will provide your body with protein:

- Boneless, skinless chicken breast;

- Skinless turkey breast or lean ground turkey;

- Egg whites;

- Lean ground meats (chicken, turkey, lamb, beef (needs to be very lean));

- Lean cuts of meat (some cuts of beef, lamb);

- Game meats (venison, bison, elk, rabbit);

- Low-fat or non-fat dairy products, such as yogurt, cottage cheese, or milk;

- Fish (tuna, salmon, mahi-mahi, orange roughy, haddock, Pollock, snapper, trout, tuna, swordfish, mackerel, halibut, sea bass, catfish, cod, flounder, etc.);

- Shellfish (shrimp, clams, crab, lobster, squid (calamari), crayfish, mussels, octopus, etc.);

- Soybean products (tofu, textured vegetable protein (TVP), soy bean curd, etc.);

- Bean Burgers (Veggie Burgers, Garden Burgers); or

- Protein powder substitute (whey, casein, egg white)

Vegetables and beans are examples of incomplete proteins because on their own they are lacking some of the essential amino acids. However, it is possible to create a complete protein by combining two foods together. For example, when you eat beans and rice or rice cakes and peanut butter. Most of the protein grams should come from complete protein sources. The best sources to choose are egg whites, chicken, turkey, white fish, tuna, salmon and whey or casein protein powder. Red meat is not easily digestible. If you choose to eat it on occasion, choose a leaner cut of meat such as a filet.

Dairy is an important component to our diet overall because it plays a part in protecting our bodies from injury and disease. It provides our bodies with the vital nutrients calcium and vitamin D. If you don't get enough of these, you will have a higher risk of developing osteoporosis. Though dairy is essential to your diet in its whole forms, it is very high in fat and calories, which is why you need to choose the fat-free or low-fat versions and consume them in moderation. Dairy should be a regular staple of your diet during maintenance periods; however, during transformation it is not the best protein choice to get you to your goals. We prefer that dairy is limited or eliminated during the transformation period, and incorporated back in during maintenance. Since it is a great source of calcium and vitamin D, please be sure to supplement with these two, or find a multi vitamin that is enriched with them as well. This is also the case if you are lactose intolerant and can't eat dairy at all.

The most important thing to remember about protein is to consume the adequate amount of protein for your fitness goals at every meal because it will help you develop, retain and increase lean muscle tissue, which in turn increases your metabolism, allowing your body to be a fat-burning machine.

Carbohydrates

With all the hype about low-carb and no-carb diets over the past few years, you (like millions of people) may believe carbohydrates are evil. We assure you that your body NEEDS carbohydrates in order to properly function. They are crucial to developing a complete nutrition plan. Carbohydrates are the preferred source of energy for your body. Without them your body can't function efficiently and effectively.

Carbs are what give us the energy to train hard, and the right types of carbs will keep you full and satisfied. They supply us with vitamins, minerals and fiber, and can be stored in our muscles and liver and utilized later for energy. They are needed for the central nervous system, kidneys, brain and muscles to function properly.

But wait! Before you head to the pantry to have a little carb indulgence, keep reading. There is some truth behind all the anti-carb hype. If you are eating the wrong type of carbs, eating them at the wrong times or eating them in higher portions than your body can utilize, they will in fact be stored very quickly in your body as fat.

Diets that completely eliminate carbohydrates are not going to be beneficial for you in the long term. The weight that you lose on a "no carb" or "super low carb" diet is mainly going to be water weight and precious lean muscle tissue. When your body is deprived of carbs, it resorts to using muscle and protein as its energy source. Essentially, your metabolism slows down and lean body mass decreases. The majority of people who have lost tons of "weight" on diets like the old Atkins plan mostly gained all their weight back and then some as soon as they caved to carb cravings, incorporated carbs back into their diets or reverted back to their old eating habits.

There are two types of carbohydrates: complex and simple. Complex carbs break down over a longer period of time and therefore, sustain us for longer periods of time. They come in two subgroups: starchy and fibrous. These are known as the "healthy carbohydrates." When you are trying to get lean, the majority of your carbohydrates will be starchy. Starchy carbs include rice, grains, potatoes, pasta and wholegrain bread. Fibrous carbs include asparagus, cauliflower, broccoli, onions and spinach and add volume to your meals without a lot of extra calories. They also contain lots of vitamins and minerals and should be incorporated into every diet.

Simple carbohydrates are simple sugars, and they don't have the nutritional value of complex carbohydrates. Sugar comes in a variety of forms, including milk, honey, chocolate, cakes, etc. This form of carbohydrate will more readily store as fat in your body. Simple carbs will spike your insulin levels which will cause them to be stored as fat. Fruits are also simple sugars, but they are a healthier option and have nutritional value due to fiber content, vitamins and minerals. The best choices for fruits are apples, raspberries, strawberries, melons and oranges. The amount of these should still be minimal, and a good diet is going to include more vegetables than fruits.

It is important to choose the right type of carbohydrates on your path towards a lean physique. The right types of carbs are going to aid you in your fat loss quest whereas the wrong ones are going to set you back and cause you to gain unwanted weight. Foods such as cookies, cakes, sodas and other sweets are high in simple carbohydrates and sugar, and will store as fat. Foods such as chips, French fries, bagels, white breads and pastas are high in carbs, and will also store as fat very easily. Avoid the non-nutritional carbs, stick with healthy carbs, and your body will be energized and will become a fat-burning machine.

Carbs are found in a wide variety of foods. Here is a list of the foods from which you should derive your carbohydrates:

Fibrous Carbs: This category encompasses your vegetables such as broccoli, Brussels sprouts, squash, spinach, tomatoes, zucchini, green beans, cauliflower, green or white asparagus, artichokes, lettuce, green/red/orange/yellow peppers, bamboo shoots, sprouts, red and green cabbage, eggplant, collard greens, onions, kale, okra, leeks, cucumbers, mushrooms, celery and Swiss chard.

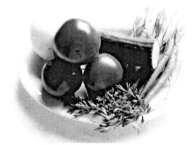

Next up are the starchy carbs. There are natural starchy carbs that haven't been processed in any way, and they are going to be your best choice for this category. They include:

- Sweet potatoes or yams;

- Beans (chick peas, black beans, black eyed peas, soy beans, butter beans, split peas, white beans, lima beans, pinto beans, navy beans, garbanzo beans, kidney beans, etc.);

- Potatoes (Red and White);

- Peas;

- Brown rice;

- Corn;

- Rye;

- Root vegetables (turnips, carrots, beets, radishes);

- Oatmeal, Cream of Wheat, Cream of Rice, Cream of Rye;

- Rye; and

- Millet.

- Butternut Squash

The next group also includes starchy carbohydrates. They are not all natural and have gone through some processing, so they aren't the number one choice, but can be used in order to offer some variety to your meals.

- Wholegrain pasta, macaroni, spaghetti;

- High fiber (low sugar) whole grain breakfast cereals;

- Muesli;

- Grits;

- Oatcakes, rice cakes;

- Shredded Wheat;

- All Bran;

- Ryvita Crisp bread;

- Corn Tortilla;

- Ezekiel Bread;

- Whole-wheat pita or tortilla;

- Low carb flat bread.

Finally, another source of natural carbohydrate includes fruits and vegetables.

Fruits and vegetables contain loads of nutrients, antioxidants and minerals, which are great for our bodies. Fruits are higher in sugar though, so during transformation periods they will be limited, but can be eaten more frequently during maintenance. It is best to have a higher intake of vegetables than fruits.

Here is a list of great vegetables and fruits that should be staples of your healthy eating program:

Veggies – (These are fibrous natural carbohydrates, when eaten in their whole forms they digest slowly and have a high thermic effect)
- Broccoli
- Asparagus
- Cauliflower
- Brussels Sprouts
- Artichokes
- Parsnips (please use in combination with other veggies, not as the main one)
- Bok Choy
- Beets (please use in combination with other veggies, not as the main one)
- Arugula
- Radishes
- Watercress
- Garlic
- Swiss Chard
- Spinach
- Zucchini
- Lettuce
- Yellow Squash
- Peppers – any kind
- Mushrooms
- Tomato
- Alfalfa or Bean Sprouts
- Bamboo Shoots
- Artichoke
- Water Chestnuts
- Cabbage
- Green Beans
- Leeks
- Okra
- Collard Greens

- Salad Greens
- Cucumbers
- Celery
- Onions
- Kale
- Carrots

Fruits:
- Apples
- Berries: Blackberries, Raspberries, Blueberries, Strawberries, Goji etc
- Cherries
- Grapefruit
- Melon: Cantaloupe, Honeydew
- Oranges
- Peaches
- Plums
- Watermelon
- Kiwi
- Papaya
- Pears
- Tangerines

Carb sources such as whole grains, vegetables, fruits and beans promote good health by delivering vitamins, minerals and fiber to the body. Fiber is an important component to your diet. We need it to stay healthy. Fiber helps maintain our gastrointestinal tract cells and without enough of it, these cells can't stay healthy, causing your body to experience deficiencies, and allow toxins to enter.

Fiber slows down the breakdown of starch and delays glucose absorption to the blood. It lowers cholesterol and helps control blood sugar levels, constipation, colon cancer, hemorrhoids, colitis and diverticulitis. You will feel more "full" when you eat foods that are higher in fiber because they take longer to chew. That "full" sensation lasts longer than if you eat foods that are low in fiber. Fiber is an important part of the equation when you are trying to lose weight, so start reading labels and choose foods that are higher in fiber. A good source of fiber will have 2.5 grams or more per serving. If you currently have little fiber in your diet, please add it in slowly. If you add it too quickly, you may experience gastrointestinal discomfort in the form of gas, diarrhea and bloating.

Next, let's discuss timing of carbohydrates. Ideally, you will be eating four to seven times per day. The meals that should contain the highest amount of carbohydrates will include your first meal of the day and your post-workout meal. A breakfast high in carbohydrates is important because your body has been fasting all night while sleeping so it needs to be refueled, and your metabolism needs to be jumpstarted for the day. Just like your mother told you, breakfast is in fact the most important meal of the day. If you skip breakfast, you are immediately sabotaging your fitness goals by putting your body into a "muscle burning" phase.

If you eliminate carbohydrates from your morning meal, you simply aren't going to be as efficient in your workouts or your daily life in general. Throughout the day, you should taper the amount of carbs you eat at each meal and avoid them (with the exception of vegetables) at your meals later in the day. The reason is that you are more active earlier in the day so your body is able to utilize the energy from the carbs throughout the day. Later at night, when your metabolism begins to slow down, carbs are not easily used for energy, so there is a much higher likelihood that they will be stored in your body as fat.

In summary, carbohydrates are not your enemy. They are an essential part of your diet and are necessary for your body to function efficiently and burn fat properly. What is most important is that you eat the right types of carbohydrates in the right portion sizes and at the right times of the day. The diet plans that are part of the Hitch Fit program are all based around these important key elements of carb consumption. Another part of what we do on the Hitch Fit online program is aid you in finding what a good carb intake level will be for you.

Sugar…Not an Essential Ingredient

Many junk foods such as cookies, chips, soda and pastries are classified as simple carbohydrates. They are typically loaded with sugar. Though all carbohydrates, even the healthy complex ones, break down into your body as sugar, the digestion rate for these simple sugar foods is much faster. When you consume carbohydrates, whether simple or complex, they break down into a simple sugar called glucose and are absorbed into your blood stream.

Your body can only handle a limited amount of sugar in the blood at one time. It is constantly trying to keep blood glucose levels stable. When you eat a high-sugar junk food that converts very quickly into blood sugar, your blood glucose levels will sky rocket quickly. To get back to balance, your body will release a hormone called insulin. The purpose of insulin is to find a place to store this extra sugar so that it doesn't stay in the blood for long periods of time. When insulin levels rise, the sugar is quickly exported from the blood. If there is no room for this sugar to be stored in muscle tissue or the liver, then it will store as fat. The more frequently you eat these types of foods, the more frequently your insulin levels are going to spike and your body will go into fat-storing mode.

The bigger the meal is, or the more junk you eat in one sitting, the more insulin your body is going to have to produce to rid the blood of all that glucose. In an unfit person especially, the majority of these calories will store as fat. Those who have had poor eating habits for long periods of time, are overweight or obese and don't exercise, can actually be at an even greater disadvantage. The constant spikes of insulin can make your muscles resistant to taking it in and storing it as glycogen for later use. Therefore, any spikes in insulin can easily transport that sugar to fat cells, so the fat can easily and readily continue to grow. This is one example of how you can continue to gain fat weight even if you under eat your calories.

Fat...the Bad

High fat foods such as fast food and fried food will lead to significant weight and fat gain easily. The reason is that fat, gram for gram is the most calorically dense nutrient. Carbohydrates are 4 calories per gram, as is protein. Fat is 9 calories per gram, so the calories will add up quickly and it is very easy to over-consume what your daily calories should be for the day.

The fats that you want to avoid are saturated fats, trans fats and hydrogenized fats. A lot of foods undergo a chemical process called hydrogenation during food processing in order to give them more flavor and a longer shelf life. It's best to limit the amount of these fats in your diet as much as possible, especially when you are trying to lose weight. These fats will not only help you gain weight, they also increase LDL levels and are the main dietary cause of high cholesterol.

Saturated fats are mostly derived from animal sources such as beef, beef fat, veal, lamb, pork, lard, poultry fat, butter, cream, milk, cheeses and other dairy products made from whole milk. They are also found in palm oil, coconut oil and palm kernel oil or cocoa butter.

When you are reading your ingredient labels, be sure to watch out for these. Trans fats (also known as partially hydrogenated fats) are found in a lot of unhealthy foods including: fried foods, crackers and cookies, any commercial snack product, vegetable oils and margarine. You should aim to keep these foods out of your diet completely. All they are going to do is hold you back from attaining your goals, and they are not good for your overall health.

If you consistently eat foods high in saturated fat, this fat goes into your blood stream clogging it up, and forcing your heart to push harder to get the blood moving through your body. This undue stress on your heart can lead to many unwanted health complications including heart attack and stroke.

Fat...the Good

Now, this doesn't mean to eliminate fats from your diet altogether. In fact, we need fat in our diets on a daily basis in order to maintain good health and to function at our highest levels. In the right portions and types, fats will actually benefit your health because they aid in cell function.

Just as with carbohydrates, the type of fats you consume, time of day, and amount that you eat are the issues that must be addressed. Being calorically higher in density, it is important to consume good fats in little amounts throughout the day with most of your meals. The time to avoid including fats in your meals is pre- and post-workout. They have a much slower digestion rate, so if you consume them around workout times your body won't be able to digest or intake the protein and carbs it needs as efficiently as possible.

Unsaturated fats are the ones that are so important for our bodies. They are the healthy fats that help us experience normal growth and development, store energy, provide cushioning for internal organs, maintain cell membranes, provide flavor, consistency and stability to our foods and help our bodies to absorb certain vitamins such as A, D, E, K and caretonoids. Healthy fats also help to lower our LDL cholesterol levels (which is the bad cholesterol that clogs up the arteries and can lead to numerous heart and healthy issues) and increase HDL levels (which is the "healthy" cholesterol). You want to have a high number of HDL. The good fats are a great source of energy for your body and will help you to avoid feeling lethargic.

There are two types of healthy fats: polyunsaturated and monounsaturated. Polyunsaturated fats have cholesterol-lowering properties. The most common types of polyunsaturated fats are Omega 3 and Omega 6. These are two essential fatty acids we must obtain from our diets because our bodies do not produce them. Most people take in more Omega 6 fatty acids, which come from plant sources, than Omega 3 fatty acids (which are also good for you and essential for health). Omega 3 fatty acids are found mostly in cold water fish, so if you aren't a big fish eater, be sure that you are attaining your Omega 3 fatty acids in supplement form.

Monounsaturated fats are also good for your heart. They are the ones that help to lower the LDL cholesterol levels. Studies show that people who eat diets higher in monounsaturated fats typically live longer and have less incidence of developing cancer. Following is a list of foods that should be used as your main source of good fats:

- Udo's Oil
- Avocado;
- Olive oil, canola oil, peanut oil, grape seed oil, fish oil;
- Olives;
- Nuts (almonds, walnuts, peanuts, cashews, macadamia and most other nuts);
- Natural peanut butter, almond butter, cashew butter, macadamia nut butter;
- Corn, soybean, safflower and other cottonseed oils;
- Fish; and
- Flax seed, hemp seed.

The most important things to remember are that healthy fats are an essential part of your diet. Eat small portions of fats throughout the day. (Your Hitch Fit diet plan will show you the amounts and times that will be best for your body and goals.) Consume mostly unsaturated fats and essential fatty acids and limit how much cheese, red meat and butter you eat. Avoid fried foods and commercial snacks. You'll satisfy your body's cravings, protect yourself from heart disease, look better and feel stronger.

Liquids

When it comes to weight loss, you have to be aware of all calories that you are ingesting in a day. That includes liquid calories! It's amazing the hundreds and even thousands of calories per day that people ingest through liquid, and they are still trying to figure out why they aren't losing fat weight. Soda and fruit juices are basically sugar in a bottle. Because the body does not fill up quickly when drinking, it is extremely easy to have your calorie intake go through the roof, even if you don't feel full. These are all simple sugars, too, so they are very easily converted into fat once consumed.

Sodas and fruit juices should be completely cut out of your diet. Some people will literally lose a couple of pounds right off the bat just by cutting out these sugary carbonated drinks. Diet sodas don't have the calories that regular soda has, but they can lead to weight gain by causing dehydration and a slow-down in your metabolism. In addition, they contain a lot of chemicals that will not allow your body to perform at optimum levels.

Another thing to be wary of is your morning caffeine kick. There's nothing wrong with a cup of coffee in the morning, but keep it straight coffee or espresso or tea. When you start getting fancy drinks with milk, whipped cream and caramel added to them, you would be amazed at how quickly the calories add up. Some of those drinks have almost 1,000 calories in them. For some people, this is more than half of what they should be consuming in an entire day! You can still drink your coffee or tea (use sugar free sweeteners such as Splenda and use skim milk instead of cream), but be sure you are drinking enough water.

Alcohol is another liquid source of empty calories that leads to weight gain. Alcohol is a drug and is stored as fat in the body because it isn't a carbohydrate and can't be metabolized by your body unless it turns it into fat. It also causes protein deficiency and dehydration. It can stimulate your appetite too; so on top of drinking empty calories, there is a good chance that you will consume excess calories, too!

We are not saying that you have to eliminate alcohol from your lifestyle forever. Personally we don't drink because we choose to give 100% to our chosen path of life, and to be walking billboards for health and fitness. If you choose to include alcohol in your life, you must practice moderation and make good choices. Don't drink on a regular basis if you are serious about achieving your fitness goals, and especially if you are undergoing transformation. If you choose to drink, stay away from drinks that are sugary. (Margaritas, daiquiris and other mixed drinks and cocktails are loaded with sugar.).

We've gone over what you shouldn't drink. What about what you should drink? The answer: water. Water is a vital element for your body to function properly. It is second only to oxygen.

You literally can't survive without water. 55 to 60% of your body weight is actually water weight. It aids in almost every basic function of your body including metabolism, temperature regulation, blood circulation and the ability of your body to flush out toxins and waste. Staying hydrated is critical to achieving your fitness goals. Having plenty of water in your body keeps your muscles full, speeds up your metabolism and helps you to feel full throughout the day, too. If you don't drink enough water, your body will actually start drawing water from the muscles themselves. Dehydration can cause fatigue and can even cause you to be moody.

Most people drink sodas and coffee and totally disregard drinking plain water. The minimum guidelines for water consumption say to drink six to eight glasses of water per day. In our opinion that is not enough. Especially since you are reading this book, indicating you are a Hitch Fit transformation in progress, or are soon to be a Hitch Fit transformation, which means you are going to be exercising regularly, sweating and needing to replenish that lost water. To figure out how much water you should be drinking, divide your body weight in pounds by two. You should be consuming a minimum of that amount in ounces of water per day. **For example, if you weigh 200 pounds you should be consuming a minimum of 100 ounces of water in a day.

Drink water consistently throughout the day even if you don't actually feel thirsty. By the time your body actually tells you that you are thirsty you are already dehydrated. Another sign that you are dehydrated is the color of your urine. If you are drinking adequate amounts of water it should be a very light yellow color. If it is a dark yellow color, drink more water.

You also need to drink just as much water in the wintertime as in the summer time. Just because it isn't hot out and you aren't sweating as much doesn't mean that you don't have to drink as much. Your body needs water in order to stay warm just as much as it does to stay cool. I would advise you to keep a record of how much water you drink as you start your transformation process. You may be amazed at how little you are drinking!

Water is the single most important beverage you should be drinking on a consistent basis throughout the day.

If you think that water is too bland, you can use lemons, limes or cucumbers to add some flavor. You can also use sugar free drink mixes such as Crystal Lite.

In conclusion, cut out the sodas and sugary drinks. Cut out or greatly moderate the amount of alcohol that you are consuming, especially during your transformation period. All of those unnecessary liquid calories are just going to hold you back from losing weight. Drink water, lots of water, every single day in order for your body to operate as efficiently as possible and in order to successfully lose weight.

The reason WHY?

The reason WHY we have our clients eat the way they do, and WHY we recommend the foods that we do in this book is because they help the body run the most efficiently. The foods that we recommend are intended to keep your blood sugar levels even and stable, thus promoting low insulin levels and production of the opposite hormone glucagon, which helps to free fat from storage in your body.

The foods that we recommend are slow digesting. They have a higher thermogenic effect, meaning the act of just eating them is burning more calories. They are the foods that are best for aiding in the maintenance and development of lean muscle tissue, which will in turn speed up your metabolism and help your body to become a fat burning machine. They are the foods that will get your body to your goals in the most efficient and effective way possible. The moral of the story here is that it isn't just about calories in versus calories out. The type of foods that you choose is also an extremely important factor if your goal is to achieve a lean and fit physique!

Timing of your calories is another important piece of the puzzle. We encourage our clients to eat small meals frequently throughout the day, and there is a reason for that. Your body can only process so many calories at one time. If you eat small meals of the right types of foods throughout the day, then your body will be able to fully utilize those calories for fuel. It will also help to keep your blood insulin levels in check all day long, and it will keep your energy levels balanced throughout the entire day.

These rules of eating apply to both transformation and maintenance. You will find that the recipes in this book are also a balance of carbohydrate, protein and fats, and will also aid in keeping blood insulin levels stable throughout the day. It's a rule that should be followed for life for optimal health and for a fit and lean physique!

HOW MANY CALORIES SHOULD YOU BE EATING IN A DAY?

This is one of the things that we help each client out with via the Hitch Fit Online Training Program. To be perfectly honest, there is no exact answer to this question. The amount of calories that we actually burn in a day varies every single day.

(***If you are not a Hitch Fit client and would like more information on the programs we have to offer please visit our website: *www.hitchfit.com*. We put the whole program together for each of our clients and take the guesswork out of the equation. We offer Lose Weight/Feel Great programs, Fitness Model and Bikini Model Programs, Muscle Building, Couples and Bridal Programs, Post Pregnancy Programs, and full Figure and Fitness Model competitor Prep programs.)

CHAPTER 2
LABELS AND TOOLS

Food Labels and Ingredient Listings

Food labels can be very misleading. Don't be fooled into thinking a product is "healthy" or good for you because it says so on the label. Just because a label says "fat free" or "sugar free" doesn't mean that is necessarily true. Labeling laws are such that as long as a serving size contains less than a certain amount of fat, sugar or calories, it can be labeled as being "free" of that product.

For example a product can be labeled as "sugar free" if it contains less than 1/2 gram of sugar per serving. Another great example is "fat-free/ calorie-free" cooking sprays. If you read the label on the back of one of these cans you will see that a serving size is 1/3 second. According to labeling laws, as long as a product has less than 1/2 gram of fat per serving it can be called "fat free," and if it has less than 5 calories per serving, it can be called "calorie free." In a full second of spray, there are actually 7 calories. If there are 702 servings in a can (1/3 second) that means that there are 234 seconds of spray in a can, which means in a "calorie free" product there are actually 1,638 calories. Cooking spray is of course a much better alternative than using butter or something heavily laden with calories. Just be aware that labels need to be looked at a little more closely and it's important to educate yourself on what the labels actually mean.

When checking out labels, you should see what the carbohydrate content, fat content and protein content are per item. See how many sugars are in the product and also check out the serving size. There are a lot of "healthy" sports drinks that contain 2 1⁄2 servings per bottle and have just as much sugar (if not more) as a bottle of soda. The same rule applies for a lot of supposedly healthy protein bars. Many of them are really high in sugar, and as you know, sugar converts to fat in your body. So, start reading the labels and if you choose to use protein bars as a supplement to your nutrition, choose the ones that are lower in sugar. A lot of these bars also contain unhealthy saturated fats and hydrogenated oils so it is a good idea to check out the ingredients list as well.

When reading an ingredient label, be aware that items are listed in the order of their prevalence. So if you pick up a product and the first ingredient is sugar or high fructose corn syrup, put it down and walk away. The same goes for products that contain trans fats and hydrogenated or partially hydrogenated products. If you are reading a label for a whole-wheat product, the first ingredient should be whole-wheat flour. If it says "enriched or bleached" it has undergone a process that has taken out most of the nutritional value.

Your Kitchen

In today's society, many people work long hours, have busy schedules, and resort to eating on the go (fast food) several times a week. You can't change your work schedule and you can't change a busy lifestyle, but you can change the way you think about food. One of the first steps in this process is to plan, and to ensure you have the proper tools.

So... you have made the decision to get "Hitch Fit". You envision pants that fit, and rocking that bathing suit. You envision being able to say... "Yes, I have had two (or more!) children" and still look like you have the metabolism of a teenager. Even the commitment to the exercise seems doable. But there is one place that even the best of us can stumble and fall if we don't properly plan for success. In order to avoid sabotaging visions of your yellow polka dot bikini, or a set of 6-pack abs to rival "The Rock", let's set some ground rules for the kitchen and get the proper tools so we experience transformation success for the long term.

The Tools

- Measuring Cups
- Measuring Spoons
- Vegetable peeler
- Good skillet
- Pyrex Baking dish
- Baking Sheet Pan
- Good knife for chopping and paring
- Cutting boards (flexible or wooden)
- Mixing Bowl
- Inexpensive Food Scale
- Non-metal, heat resistant spatula
- Tupperware or Glad ware
- Shaker Bottles
- Mini Cooler for when you are traveling
- Blender

Herbs & Spices

Don't be afraid to spice up your foods! Herbs and Spices are a great low or no calorie way to add variety too. In addition to the recipe ideas in this book, you can try out any of the spices below to season your foods and find combinations that you enjoy! They add great variety of flavor to your food for very little or no calories. They are sold in ground and whole forms. The whole form of herbs and spices is best. You can grind them yourself in a coffee grinder. However, pre-ground versions are also fine.

The following spices or ingredients are a partial list, but there are many other spices you can use, and they are great staples to keep on the shelf:

Spices

Allspice: Spicy in flavor, ground version is best, great on salads or in oatmeal;
Anise: Sweet flavor, dried seeds, good on chicken;
Basil: Slightly sweet, fresh leaves are best, good with tomatoes, eggplant, or good addition to salads;
Black Pepper: Slightly hot flavor, best ground, add to any dish to give a little heat;
Borage : Mild flavor, adds flavor to salads;
Capers: Pickled, can be used in salads;
Caraway: Sweet, nutty flavor;
Cardamom: Sweet spicy flavor, use whole or ground, don't use too much it is very strong;
Cayenne Pepper: Very hot, dried, ground or fresh, can use on meats, vegetables, eggs, anything that you would like a hot spicy flavor with;
Celery Seed: Celery flavor, whole seed, can use in cooking meats or add to salads;
Chervil: Similar to parsley, can be used in salads or on omelet's;
Chile Powder: Very spicy and hot, use on anything you would like to add some spice and heat to;
Chives: onion and garlic type flavor, best fresh, can add to salads or use as garnish;
Cilantro: spicy, sweet and hot, can be used in omelet's, salads, salsas;
Cinnamon: Sweet, can be used in shakes or oatmeal;
Cloves: sweet to bittersweet flavor;
Coriander: spicy, sweet or hot flavor, use ground or whole;
Cumin: Peppery flavor, don't use too much, very strong flavor;
Curry Powder: Spicy and hot;
Dill: mild and slightly sour taste, good for fish, eggs, potatoes, meats, salads;
Fennel: Licorice flavor, good for salads;
Fenugreek: sweet flavor, can be good for meat dishes;
Garlic: mildly hot, pungent flavor, use sparingly, salads, meats etc. can use ground or fresh variety;
Ginger: Peppery and sweet, good for adding into oats or shakes;

Green Peppercorns: Mild, sweet;
Horseradish: Condiment for fish, beef, potato, very sharp flavor;
Mint: Many varieties of mint, great with salads and vegetables or as tea;
Mustard: Several varieties, some milder than others, good on meats, fish, salads;
Nutmeg: sweet and spicy, good for adding to shakes and oats;
Oregano: Slightly sweet, good with veggies;
Paprika: sweet to hot flavor, good with potato, eggs, salads;
Parsley: mild pepper flavor, used as garnish or in salads;
Poppy Seed: nutty flavor, good for salads or oats;
Rosemary: lemon and piney flavor, great for fish and meat;
Saffron: pungent, used in rice and fish (very expensive);
Sage: A slight bitter flavor, good with beef and fish and common for turkey;
Salt: Sea salt is best, use moderately, can be used on wide variety of foods;
Sesame Seed: Nutty flavor, salads or fish;
Summer Savory: milder minty flavor, good for beans, fish, meat dishes, it is strong so use sparingly;
Tarragon: tastes like Anise, good with eggs and seafood;
Thyme: Mint and lemony, good in omelet's, chicken, salads and cooked veggies;
Turmeric: slightly bitter, kind of like ginger, good for spicy flavors;
Vanilla: sweet flavor, good in coffee or even in shakes;
White Pepper: milder than black pepper, add to foods for some heat;
Winter Savory: tastes like combo of mint and thyme, good on meat, fish and bean dishes.

Great spices to use to help boost your metabolism are:
Ginger (add a sprinkle to your oatmeal or in shakes, can boost metabolism up to 20% for 3 hours after eating);
Mustard spice or seed (add to chicken, turkey, fish or salads, this can also boost metabolism up to 20% for a couple hours after);
Cayenne Pepper – If you can handle the heat this has also been proven to boost metabolism for a couple hours post consumption, add to salads, chicken, turkey etc.

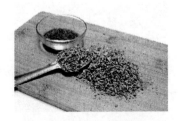

Chapter 3

Healthy Egg Recipes

*All Nutritional Values provided in these recipes may vary according to size of eggs, brand you choose and portion sizes. Please be diligent about reading your labels and nutritional information. What it says on the label of the product you choose always trumps general guidelines!

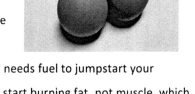

Skipping breakfast isn't unusual these days. Breakfast, in many people's eyes, is the least important meal of the day and is often given the least attention. This can't be further from the truth. Your body has been starving all night and needs fuel to jumpstart your metabolism for the day. You want your body to start burning fat, not muscle, which is what happens if you don't feed your body.

What You Should Not Be Eating For Breakfast...

If you are trying to lose weight it is obviously best to avoid foods high in saturated fat and calories. Even if you are not on a diet, greasy foods or sugary cereal are not the most sensible or the healthiest choice. Your breakfast should include fiber and protein, so oatmeal with a scoop of good whey protein isolate would be an excellent choice. A fruit smoothie is also a quick and nutritious drink, especially good if you're on the go. There really is no excuse for not eating breakfast.

About Eggs:

Here are some of the forms you will find eggs in:

Eggs Whites

If you want all the benefits of eggs without the fat, then remove the yolk from your eggs and only cook using the whites. The average egg white contains less than twenty calories! Egg whites are rich in vitamins and protein, and can be used in exactly the same way as whole eggs.

Egg Substitute

Egg substitute is an excellent alternative to whole eggs and can be found in most supermarkets. It is made of fresh or powdered egg whites. Egg substitute is quick and easy. All you have to do is pour the right amount into the skillet, stir and serve. It is low in calories and cholesterol while still retaining much of the nutritional value  of whole eggs.

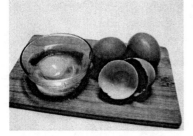

Whole Eggs

Whole eggs are full of flavor and are excellent for any meal of the day. They are incredibly versatile and full of essential nutrients. A whole egg contains 75 calories, 6 g of protein and 5 g of fat.

They are suitable for the whole family, and can be eaten by both vegetarians and lactose intolerant alike. It is also easy to add one whole egg into egg whites to add flavor and depth without adding the fat of more than one egg.

EGG WHITE OMELETS

Spinach Sprinkled Egg White Omelet

Ingredients:

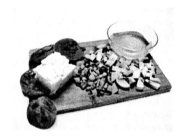

3 egg whites
1 tablespoon of water
½ teaspoon dried mixed herbs (Italian
Blend)
Freshly ground black pepper (to taste)
¾ cups chopped fresh baby spinach
*1 oz. low-fat or fat-free shredded sharp
cheddar or grated Parmesan (*maintenance phase only)
Olive Oil Cooking Spray

Instructions:

First gather your ingredients and tools. You will need a non-stick skillet, mixing bowl, and spatula.

In a bowl, combine the 3 egg whites, water and herbs. Beat together until thoroughly mixed. Lightly coat a nonstick skillet with olive oil spray. Place the oiled skillet over medium heat. Add the fresh baby spinach to the skillet. When the spinach starts to cook; the spinach will begin to wilt; pour the egg mixture over the spinach. When the edges of the egg have set, gently lift the egg from the pan to ensure the entire omelet is being cooked through and is not burning or sticking to the skillet. When the egg whites are fully cooked, add cheese to the top and fold the omelet over. *Only add cheese if you are in the maintenance phase. **Add salt and pepper to taste.

**Tip and Suggestions: Add your favorite herb mixture or you may substitute the dried herbs for fresh in twice the amount. Don't be afraid to play with the herbs or spices used... adding some paprika for color would be great on top of this omelet. Spices add depth without calories!

Cooking time (duration): 10 minutes; Serves: 1; Nutritional value per serving: Calories: 146; Fat 6.1 g (sat 3.5 g); Cholesterol 20 mg; Carbohydrate 0.8 g; Fiber 0.5 g; Protein 19.6 g.

Summer Garden Omelet

Summer veggies are beautiful in the garden but they're even more appealing on a plate. This omelet incorporates your favorite summer veggies to create a hearty breakfast to get you going. So, when it's time to harvest your garden or you just want a touch of summer, this omelet is surely the way to go.

Ingredients:

   1/3 cup sliced or diced red, green or yellow bell pepper
   ½ cup chopped zucchini
   1-2 tablespoons chopped green onions
   ½ cup halved cherry tomatoes
   ¼ teaspoon salt, divided
   2 tablespoons water
   ¼ teaspoon black pepper
   3 large egg whites
   1 large whole egg
   *2 tablespoons shredded low-fat Gouda cheese or low-fat mozzarella
   (*Maintenance phase only)

Instructions:

Add 1 to 2 tablespoons olive oil to a saucepan. Sauté peppers, zucchini, onions and 1/8-teaspoon salt until veggies are slightly tender but still crisp. They should still have bright, vibrant color. Take the saucepan from the heat and set aside.

In a bowl, mix remaining salt, water, egg whites and egg. Spray a 10" skillet with olive oil cooking spray and heat. Add egg mixture to pan and let cook until the edges set. Lift to ensure that no raw egg remains in the pan.

Scoop veggie mix onto omelet and *cover with cheese then fold in half. Cook until cheese melts. Salt and pepper to taste.

Cooking time (duration): 20 minutes; Serves: 1; Nutritional value per serving: 252 Calories; Fat 12.9g (sat 6.5g); Sodium 476 mg; Carbohydrate 9.8g; Fiber 3g; Protein 26.4g.

South of the Border Omelet

A little spice can surely jump start your day. This omelet gives you just the kick you need with green chilies and picante sauce. You don't have to go south of the border to enjoy robust flavors. Use this recipe to bring the vibrant flavors of the south to you.

Ingredients:

> 3 egg whites, beaten
> ½ cup water
> ¼ teaspoon salt
> ¼ cup green chilies
> ¼ cup finely chopped onion
> ¼ teaspoon chili powder
> 1/8 teaspoon ground cumin
> 1-2 tablespoons olive oil (Or Olive Oil Cooking Spray for less calories)
> *1/4 cup shredded low fat or fat-free Monterey Jack or Mexican blend cheese (*Only during maintenance phase)
> 3 tablespoons Picante sauce or salsa (*Be careful to read the ingredients, as some jarred salsa contains added sugar and lots of sodium. Approximately 300 g of sodium are included below in the nutritional information with 3 tablespoons of traditional Picante.)

Instructions:

In a bowl, combine eggs, water, salt and spices. Pour in onions and chilies and stir together. *If desired, you could also sauté the onions and chilies together with 1 tablespoon of olive oil first to soften them prior to adding them in with the egg mixture.

Lightly spray a skillet with olive oil spray or 1 tablespoon of olive oil. Slowly rotate the pan to coat. Pour in the egg mixture. When the edges are set, slightly lift so the eggs don't stick and so the entire mixture cooks evenly.

When the egg whites set, add ½ of the cheese. When it is cooked through, fold over, and add remainder of cheese. Remove from the skillet and top with picante sauce if desired. (Cheese during the maintenance phase only).

*Tips and Suggestions: A fresh salsa can be made using onion, green peppers, chilies and tomatoes. Add freshly ground pepper to taste.

Cooking time (duration): 20 minutes; Serves: 1; Nutritional value per serving: 257 calories; Fat 16.8 g (sat 3.3 g); Sodium 621 mg; Carbohydrate 7.5 g; Fiber 1.3 g; Protein 20.3 g.

Mushroom, Spinach and Feta Omelet

Veggies are a terrific way to get the vitamins and nutrients that you need daily. Getting a serving with your morning meal is an ideal way to start. This recipe uses spinach and mushrooms to fill you up and give you a boost of your daily nutritional requirements.

Ingredients:

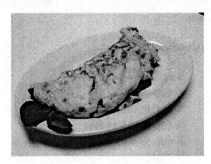

1 whole egg
3 egg whites
*2 tablespoons low-fat or fat-free Feta Cheese (*maintenance phase only)
¼ teaspoon salt
1/8 teaspoon crushed red pepper flakes
1/8 teaspoon garlic powder
1/8 teaspoon pepper
½ cup sliced fresh mushrooms
2 tablespoons finely chopped red onion
1 tablespoon olive oil
1 cup torn spinach

Instructions:

Beat egg and egg whites together in a bowl. Mix in cheese and seasonings. Sauté vegetables with olive oil (or use PAM cooking spray for less calories and fat) in a nonstick skillet until they are tender. Add spinach and cook until the spinach begins to wilt.

Pour egg mixture over vegetables and cook. Slice omelet into sections and serve immediately.

*Tips and Suggestions: Don't be afraid to try a dash of hot sauce to liven it up!

Cooking time (duration): 20 minutes

Serves: 2 Nutritional value per serving: 164 Calories; Fat 11.7g (sat 3.0g); Sodium 616mg; Carbohydrate 2.4g; Fiber 0.8g; Protein 13.3g.

Calories based on 2 equal portions of ingredients.

Turkey & Vegetable Omelet

Omelets are a unique dish. They can be made with anything you like. This omelet combines turkey bacon and vegetables to create a dish packed with flavor and color. Easy to make and filling, let this dish brighten up your day before it really gets started.

Ingredients:

   3 slices Jennie O extra lean turkey bacon
   1 tablespoon minced garlic
   1 tablespoon minced onion
   ¼ cup diced green bell pepper
   ¼ cup diced red bell pepper
   ¼ diced yellow bell pepper
   ¼ cup broccoli, precooked, and small dice
   1 tablespoon chopped basil
   1 tablespoon fresh parsley
   1 whole egg
   3 egg whites
   *¼ cup shredded low-fat Cheddar Cheese (*Maintenance phase only)
   **Season with salt and pepper and chives to taste

Instructions:

Cook bacon over medium heat in a nonstick skillet until the bacon begins to cook through to the desired consistency. Pour in the garlic and onions and continue to cook for about 2 minutes (they will start to become transparent). Stir in the rest of the vegetables and cook until peppers start to get soft. Remove ingredients from skillet. Crumble bacon and add back to the dish.

Beat eggs together and add salt and pepper. Pour eggs into skillet and cook until edges begin to set. Flip the egg over and back quickly to ensure that all egg is cooked. Place cheese and vegetable mixture down the middle of the egg. Fold each side in to the center.

*Tips and Suggestion: Serve this omelet with salsa and sprinkle with chives.

Cooking time (duration): 1 hour

Serves: 2; Nutritional value per serving: 187 Calories; Fat 7.8g (sat 3.0g); Sodium 796mg; Carbohydrate 9.7g; Fiber 3.2g; Protein 19.3g.

Calories based on 2 equal portions of ingredients.

The Good morning Succotash Omelet (Egg Whites)

Ingredients:

- 1 tablespoon olive oil (Or Olive Oil Cooking Spray)
- 1 bag of frozen mixed vegetables (unthawed)
- ½ teaspoon dried thyme (or 1 teaspoon fresh chopped thyme)
- ½ teaspoon cayenne pepper
- 4 egg whites
- *1 oz of low-fat cheddar (*maintenance phase only)

Instructions:

In a skillet, heat olive oil in a non-stick pan and add frozen vegetable medley, herbs and seasonings.

Cook until the vegetables are fork tender. Transfer the vegetable mixture to a bowl and return the skillet to medium heat. Pour in the egg whites and let cook until the edges are beginning to cook through. Add the vegetable mixture and top with low-fat cheddar shred, fold over and serve.

Serves: 2 Nutritional value per serving: 211 Calories; Fat 8.8g (sat 1.8g); Sodium 264mg; Carbohydrate 19.7g; Fiber 5.9g; Protein 16.3g.

Calories based on 2 equal portions of ingredients.

Love in the Morning Casserole

Everyone needs a little love to start the day. This breakfast casserole, with artichoke hearts as its main ingredient, will fill your heart and your stomach. So, use this easy recipe to get your day started off with a touch of love.

Ingredients:

13 oz. can of artichoke hearts
½ medium red onion, finely chopped
½ cup of mushrooms, sliced
½ cup sweet corn
2 cloves garlic, finely chopped
1 1/3 cup egg substitute like Egg Beaters (equates to about 5 ½ egg whites)
½ cup uncooked old-fashioned oatmeal (pulsed in a blender to give it the consistency of bread crumbs) (**could also use ¼ Panko crumbs in maintenance phase)
¼ teaspoon salt
¼ teaspoon pepper
¼ teaspoon dried oregano
½ teaspoon cayenne pepper
*1 cup low fat shredded cheddar cheese (*maintenance phase only)

Instructions:

To start, turn the oven to 325 degrees to preheat. Pour the juice from the artichoke can into a skillet, straining and reserving the artichokes. Chop artichokes and put them in a bowl to the side. Heat the artichoke juice over medium heat and simmer. Add the onions, mushrooms and corn to the skillet and sauté for 5 minutes.

In a bowl, place egg substitute and add oatmeal, salt, pepper, oregano and cayenne pepper. Add cheese, chopped artichokes and skillet contents to the bowl. Mix thoroughly.

Coat a "7x11" casserole dish with a thin spray of olive oil. Bake for half an hour, or until the egg is set all the way through. Cut and serve.

*Tips and Suggestions: The cayenne pepper in this recipe can be substituted by Tabasco sauce or jalapeno pepper.

Serves: 6 Nutritional values per serving: 163 Calories; Fat 6.4 g (sat 0.9 g); Cholesterol 8mg; Sodium 447mg; Carbohydrate 16.4 g; Fiber 1.4 g; Protein 11.4 g.

Calories based on 6 equal portions of ingredients.

Turkey to Go Skillet

Breakfast on the move is easy with this turkey bacon breakfast in a skillet. Filled with your favorite breakfast foods, bacon and eggs, you'll be satisfied with just one. When you have to move and move fast, take your turkey bacon to go!

Ingredients :

    5 slices Jennie O's extra lean turkey bacon
    ½ cup green pepper, chopped
    ½ cup onion, chopped
    5 whole eggs or 1¼ cups egg substitute
    ½ cup low-fat milk
    ¼ teaspoon black pepper
    *1 cup reduced fat (or Kraft Free) cheddar cheese, grated (*maintenance phase only)

Instructions :

Clean all cooking surfaces and utensils before you begin.

Cook bacon, green pepper and onion for 12-15 minutes in a large skillet over medium heat. Stir often and cook until bacon is nicely browned. Take skillet off heat.

In a separate bowl, mix eggs, milk and pepper. Blend well. Pour egg mixture into skillet on top of bacon mixture. Cook over low heat until eggs are almost done and remove from heat. Stir in cheese.

*Tips and Suggestions: Make an all-natural salsa with chopped tomatoes, onion and green pepper. For a sweet addition, try chopped mango. You can also add all your favorite veggies and spice the dish to your desired tastes.

Cooking time (duration): 30 minutes

Serves: 4 Nutritional values per serving: 189 Calories; Fat 7.5 (sat 2.3g); Sodium 556 mg; Carbohydrate 6.5g; Fiber 0.6 g; Protein 21.9 g.

Calories based on 4 equal portions of ingredients.

Tex-Mex Egg White Scramble

Tired of plain old scrambled egg whites? Add some color, spice and recreate a morning original with a zesty taste.

Ingredients:

1 lb. of lean ground turkey
    ½ teaspoon ground cumin
    ½ teaspoon dried oregano
    1 teaspoon of chili powder
    ½ cup "no salt added" diced tomatoes
    1 small Spanish onion, finely diced
    1/2 green, yellow or red bell pepper, finely diced
    ¼ cup of canned, chopped green chilies
    1 whole egg
    4 egg whites (1 cup)
    ¼ cup of fat free mozzarella cheese (*During maintenance phase)

Instructions :

First, gather your ingredients and tools. Place the ground turkey in a large, deep skillet. Cover and cook over medium-high heat for a few minutes, and then add the onion, pepper and chilies. Cook until the turkey is evenly brown and the vegetables are soft. While the turkey and veggies are cooking, beat the egg and egg whites together in a bowl. Mix in cheeses and seasonings. Pour egg mixture over vegetables and turkey and cook through. Slice into sections and serve immediately.

Serves: 4 Nutritional values per serving: 255 Calories; Fat 9.6g (sat 2.9g); Sodium 537mg; Carbohydrate 9.8g; Fiber 2.0g; Protein 31.4g.

Calories based on 4 equal portions of ingredients.

Zany Zu-corn Mini Quiche

*Maintenance phase recipe

Eating healthy doesn't have to be boring. No one wants to eat the same things for breakfast all of the time. Sometimes, change is good. Well, this recipe can definitely put a zany spin to breakfast. This easy to make recipe will have you singing its praises with just one bite.

Ingredients :

3 large whole eggs
3 large egg whites
½ teaspoons baking powder
1 medium zucchini, finely diced
½ medium yellow onion, finely diced
¼ medium green bell pepper, diced
½ cup frozen yellow sweet corn
3 oz. low-fat feta cheese, crumbled
2 tablespoons low-fat Parmesan cheese, grated

Instructions :

Before you start, make sure that all of your cooking surfaces and utensils are clean and ready to be used.

Turn the oven on and preheat at 350 degrees.

Cook zucchini, onion, peppers and corn in a pan at medium heat until the onion becomes transparent. Approximately 5 minutes and let sit until it cools slightly.

In a bowl, mix whole eggs, egg whites, cheese and baking powder. Feel free to use a hand mixer if one is accessible. The mixture is done when it's creamy.

Add cooked, and cooled zucchini mixture into the liquid mixture and mix well. *Make sure it has cooled slightly so it doesn't start cooking the egg mixture when it is stirred in. Use ¼-cup measuring cup to pour batter into silicone cupcake pans and bake. The cupcakes should be done in about 20-25 minutes. The center should be set.

*Tips and Suggestions: Check doneness with a toothpick by inserting the toothpick into the center of the quiche. If the toothpick comes out clean, they're done. If batter is on the toothpick, bake an additional 5-10 minutes. This mini quiche can be stored in the refrigerator. Try adding lean turkey bacon for another layer of flavor.

Cooking time (duration): 35 minutes

Serves: 12 Nutritional values per serving: 54 Calories; Fat 2.6g (sat 0.9g); Cholesterol 5mg; Sodium 214 mg; Carbohydrate 3.3g; Fiber 0.6g; Protein 4.9g.

Calories based on 12 equal portions of ingredients.

Mushroom and Tomato Egg Skillet

This could be called the breakfast of champions, loaded with all the nutritional ingredients your body needs to begin the day.

Ingredients:

- 1 tablespoon olive oil (or cooking spray)
- 6 ounces of button mushrooms (thinly diced) about 2 cups.
- 1 medium tomato, chopped. (You can substitute canned tomatoes.)
- 1 teaspoon dried thyme
- ½ teaspoon rosemary
- ½ teaspoon freshly ground black pepper
- 1 cup frozen sliced Zucchini
- 1 1/2 cups of egg substitute or 6 egg whites.

Instructions:

Heat olive oil in a non-stick skillet over medium heat; add mushrooms, stir as needed. Cook until mushrooms release their natural liquid, add tomatoes, zucchini, and dried herbs. After 2 or 3 minutes, once the zucchini starts to soften, pour in egg mixture and cook through. This can either be a scrambled egg mixture or let it set through and flip the sides up to form an omelet.

Serves 2 Nutritional values per serving: 194 Calories; 21.3g Protein; 10.3 g Carbohydrates; 3.0 g Fiber; Fat 7.3 g; Sodium 356 mg.

Calories based on 2 equal portions of ingredients.

Portabella Mushroom Morning Delight

*Maintenance Phase Recipe

Mushrooms are good with any meal, but they usually play a supporting role. If you're in the market for an elegant, yet healthy breakfast dish, try this breakfast casserole. Portabella mushrooms are the featured stars of this sophisticated entrée. You'll never look at mushrooms the same way again.

This dish requires refrigeration for at least 2 hours prior to cooking

Ingredients:

2 cups portabella mushrooms (chopped)

2 cloves garlic (minced)

½ cup red onions (sliced)

1 teaspoon rosemary (chopped)

2 slices whole wheat bread, sprouted grain or Ezekiel bread (cut into small cubes) *(Or you could substitute ½ cup oatmeal)

4 oz. low-fat cheddar cheese (finely grated)

8 whole eggs (or 2 cups egg substitute)

1 cup nonfat milk

½ teaspoon salt

½ teaspoon pepper

Olive oil cooking spray (PAM)

Instructions:

Lightly coat frying pan with Olive Oil cooking spray (PAM) and place over medium heat. Sauté mushrooms, garlic, onion and rosemary until the vegetables are tender, but not cooked all the way.

Coat a casserole dish, the ideal dish for this recipe would be 1.5 qt. or 8" round, with a very light coat of olive oil spray. Evenly place half of the bread cubes into the dish. On top of the bread, in layers, place half the cheese and half the sautéed vegetable mixture. Do this until all of the ingredients are used.

In another bowl, combine the eggs, milk, salt and pepper. Pour the liquid ingredients over the contents of the casserole dish and cover the dish with plastic wrap. Put the dish in the refrigerator for at least 2 hours or overnight.

When you are ready to cook, bake the casserole in a 350-degree oven for at least 45 minutes or until the center of the casserole is set. Let the hot casserole sit for at least 5 minutes before serving.

*Tips and Suggestions: Add various herbs to this recipe to create more layers of flavor. This dish is best served hot. If you opt for egg whites, and oatmeal instead of breadcrumbs, this recipe could be used during your initial or transformation phase.

Cooking time (duration): 1 hour and 15 minutes

Serves: 4 Nutritional values per serving: 295 Calories; Fat 10.6g (sat 2.5g); Sodium 523 mg; Carbohydrate 24.3; Fiber 3.6g; Protein 26.1g.

Calories based on 4 equal portions of ingredients.

CHAPTER 4

MORE BREAKFAST RECIPES!

Note: Many of these breakfast recipes would serve as your carbohydrate source in the morning. You will want to have them alongside a protein power source such as eggs or egg whites; whey protein isolate powder; or lean turkey bacon for a complete meal. Read your labels to find out the additional calories and macronutrients that these additions will add.

All Nutritional Values provided in these recipes may vary according to the brand you choose and portion sizes. Please still be diligent about reading your labels and nutritional information. What it says on the label of the product you choose always trumps general guidelines!

Browned Cinnamon Eggplant

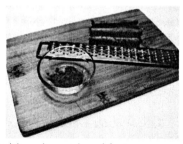

Breakfast ingredients aren't written in stone and rules were made to be broken anyway. Bread isn't the only thing that makes a great French toast breakfast. This recipe, using eggplant, is a healthy alternative to the sweet breakfast everyone loves to indulge in. Don't cheat yourself. Use this easy recipe and put a healthy edge on breakfast.

Ingredients:

1 small eggplant
1 egg white
1 tablespoon cinnamon
1/8 teaspoon nutmeg
1 Packet of Stevia or Truvia
Olive Oil Spray (PAM)

Instructions:

Prior to cooking in your kitchen, be sure that all of your surfaces and cooking utensils are clean.

Start by cutting the small eggplant into disks that are ¼ - ½" thick. In a bowl, mix egg white, cinnamon, nutmeg and Stevia. Place the eggplant into the mixture and allow a few minutes for it to soak. Lightly spray pan with Olive Oil spray or PAM. Brown the eggplant on both sides, in a pan over medium heat.

*Tips and suggestions: You can use fruit as toppings. This dish should be prepared and eaten immediately. This meal meets carb and fat requirements, please eat with a protein source such as eggs or lean turkey bacon.

Cooking time (duration): 15 minutes; Serves: 2 Nutritional values per serving: 150 Calories; Fat 7.7 (sat 1.2g); Sodium 36.6 mg; Carbohydrate 19.9g; Fiber 8.8 g; Protein 4.9g.

Calories based on 2 equal portions of ingredients.

Tasty Tofu French Banana Toast With Berries
(*Maintenance phase)

Who said you can't have French toast when you're trying to lose weight. Tofu can make a lot of things possible. Try this recipe for Tasty Tofu French Banana Toast and enjoy the start of your day again!

Ingredients:

    3 slices whole wheat bread or Ezekiel or spelt bread
    1 banana (ripe)
    8 oz. Silken Lite Firm Tofu
    1-2 teaspoon vegetable oil (may need to add a little more oil between batches so bread doesn't burn)
    ¾ cup 1% milk or soy milk
    ½ teaspoon vanilla or almond extract
    1 teaspoon cinnamon

Instructions:

Be sure that all of your cooking utensils and surfaces are clean before you begin cooking.

In a bowl, mix all of the ingredients except for the bread and vegetable oil. Mix them until they have the consistency of a batter. You can use a blender to mix the ingredients and pour the batter into a bowl.

Preheat the skillet over low to medium heat for 1 minute, and then add a very light coat of vegetable oil. If you are using a pan that isn't nonstick, coat it enough so that the battered bread won't stick.

When the oil is heated, dip a slice of bread into the batter and place it flat on the skillet's bottom. When the bottom side of the bread has reached the desired shade of brown, flip the bread to achieve the same color on the other side. Do this with all 3 slices. Serve immediately.

*Tips and Suggestions: Try adding a pinch of nutmeg to the recipe as well; it will add another layer of flavor without calories. You can substitute the low-fat milk in this recipe for soymilk. Also, you can slice the bread into strips, making French toast sticks instead. *Top with fresh berries and nuts to add flavor. This has some protein from tofu, but if you have it alongside eggs, turkey bacon or a protein shake, it is a more complete meal.

Cooking time (duration): 15 minutes; Serves: 3 Nutritional values per serving: 246 Calories; Fat 6.2g (sat 2.6 g); Sodium 252 mg; Carbohydrate 37.6 g; Fiber 4.2 g; Protein 11.1 g.

Calories based on 3 equal portions of ingredients.

Butternut Squash Hash browns

Hash browns have always been a breakfast staple, but when you're dieting, you try to limit how many starchy carbohydrates you eat.

This is a simple alternative for you to enjoy in place of conventional hash browns. In a few minutes, you can enjoy a hearty breakfast that's full of flavor...just add some egg whites and it's a complete meal.

Ingredients:

1 cup shredded butternut squash

1-2 tablespoons olive oil

2 tablespoons onions chopped

¼ teaspoon garlic powder

¼ teaspoon onion powder

Dash of cumin

Dash of salt

Dash of pepper

*Season to Taste

Instructions:

Always clean your cooking surfaces and utensils before you start cooking.

Use a couple of paper towels to absorb as much moisture as you can from the squash. Toss the shredded squash with the seasonings. Use 1 or 2 tablespoons of olive oil to lightly coat a medium pan. Place pan over medium heat. Once pan is hot, add shredded squash mixture and cook until squash is golden brown on all sides.

*Tips and suggestions: Squash tends to retain water so it's important that you remove as much water as possible before cooking it. Add Bell pepper and low fat cheese for additional flavor. This is a carb source, so eat along with protein such as eggs, turkey bacon or a protein shake for a complete breakfast.

Cooking time (duration) 8 minutes; Serves: 1 Nutritional value per serving: 116 Calories; Fat 0.4 g (sat 0.0 g); Sodium 169 mg; Carbohydrate 29.2 g; Fiber 6.9 g; Protein 2.9 g.

Calories based on 1 portion of ingredients.

Tofu & Mushroom Breakfast Scramble

Enjoy breakfast without all the added calories. This simple tofu breakfast is loaded with flavor and is just as mouth-watering as it looks.

Ingredients:

1/2 cup yellow onion, diced

1/2 cup green bell pepper, diced

¼ cup diced mushrooms

1/2 block tofu, drained and pressed

1 tablespoon olive oil

1 teaspoon garlic powder

1 teaspoon onion powder

2 teaspoons lite soy sauce

2 tablespoon Red star nutritional yeast powder

1/2 teaspoon turmeric (optional)

Instructions:

Slice the tofu into one-inch cubes; and crumble with a fork. Heat a skillet for 1 minute and then add the olive oil. When the oil is hot, add the onions, peppers and mushrooms and sauté for 2 or 3 minutes, until veggies start to soften. Add crumbled tofu to the veggie mixture for 3-5 minutes, stirring often. Add remaining ingredients, reduce heat to medium and cook 5-7 more minutes, stirring frequently and adding water for moisture if needed.

*Tips and Suggestions: *During maintenance phase, wrap tofu breakfast in a warm wheat tortilla shell and top with homemade salsa for a spicy kick.

Serves 1: Nutritional Values per serving: Calories: 387; Fat: 29.4 g (4.4 g sat. fat); Carbohydrates: 31 g; Fiber: 10.7 g; Protein: 37.3 g; Sugar: 4.1 g.

Calories based on 1 portion of ingredients.

Peanut Butter Cup Cream of Wheat

Chocolate and peanut butter flavors are a great duo and delicious when combined! But you do have to be careful with this combo as calories can add up if you over do it!

Ingredients:

1 ¼ cups water

¼ cup Cream of Wheat (with or without salt)

1 serving Jell-O-brand Fat Free, Sugar Free Chocolate Pudding

1 tablespoon natural, creamy peanut butter – OR for a lower calorie version with maximum flavor use PB2 peanut butter flavoring!

Instructions:

In a small saucepan, add cream of wheat to water and cook for 60 seconds. Stir the mixture and cook for another 60 seconds.

Mix peanut butter (or PB2) and pudding into the saucepan. Cook for 60 seconds while stirring. Serve while hot.

*Tips and Suggestions: No sweeteners are needed in this recipe, the pudding is enough. This meal serves as carb and fat requirements. Stir in one scoop of whey protein isolate for a protein source, try a chocolate or vanilla flavor. Or eat this alongside egg whites or turkey bacon.

Serves: 1 Nutritional Values: 192 Calories per serving. Total Fat: 8.4 g (1.9 g sat), Total Carbs: 19.1 g, Protein: 5.1g, Fiber: 2.3g

Raisin-Apple Cream of Barley

This recipe is simple and flavorful. Kick start your morning with this warm and savory breakfast cereal.

Ingredients:

  1 cup medium pearled barley
  1 cup unsweetened applesauce
  ½ cup raisins
  1 tablespoon Stevia or 1 packet Truvia
  1 teaspoon cinnamon
  6 cups water

Instructions:

Be sure that all of your cooking surfaces and utensils are clean prior to cooking.

Bring 6 cups water to a brisk boil over medium heat in a medium sized saucepan. Add all ingredients to boiling water. Cover the saucepan with a fitted lid and lower the heat. Let ingredients simmer until tender.

Remove saucepan from heat and let stand for 5 minutes.

*Tips and Suggestions: To reheat, add a small amount of low-fat milk and stir over low heat. Also, Craisins or other dried fruit can be substituted for the raisins, or omit fruit entirely to lower carbohydrate and sugar content of the dish. Nutmeg or allspice can be substituted for cinnamon. This meal is a carb source, so stir in a scoop of whey protein isolate or eat alongside egg whites or turkey bacon for a complete meal.

Cooking time (duration): 1 hour and 5 minutes

Serves: 4 Nutritional Value: Calories per serving: 266g; Total Fat: 0.7 g (0.2 g sat fat), Total Carbs: 62.7 g, Protein: 5.7 g

Calories based on 4 equal portions of ingredients.

Mexican Bean Breakfast

Beans, beans, good for your heart! Give your day a healthy start! This recipe uses healthy lentil beans to create a savory breakfast cereal like you have never tasted before. A sweet breakfast isn't always what you want. Here's an alternative that will surely leave a good impression.

Ingredients:

    ½ cup dried lentils
    2 cups low sodium chicken broth
    ¼ cup prepared salsa (recipe below)
    2 cups fresh spinach
    Salsa (or Newman's Own, 3 tablespoons)
    ½ cup chopped tomato
    ½ cup chopped green pepper
    ¼ cup chopped onion
    ¼ chopped mango (optional – exclude to reduce sugars)

Instructions:

Clean all work surfaces and cooking utensils before cooking.

In a saucepan, bring chicken broth and lentils to a slow boil.

Once boiling, immediately reduce heat to a simmer. Simmer until lentils are tender (approximately 15-20 minutes). Add spinach and let cook until just wilted. Remove from heat immediately. Add salsa and seasoning to taste.

*Tips and Suggestion: Adding tomatoes to beans will cause the skin of the beans to become tough, so it's important to wait to add salsa until the pan is removed from the heat. You are receiving protein from your beans, but for added protein, include a side of egg whites or a protein shake.

Cooking time (duration): 22 minutes; Serves: 1 Nutritional Values: Calories per serving: 170g; Total Fat: 0.8 g, (0.1 g sat); Total Carbs: 26.3 g; Protein: 15.6 g; Fiber: 10.6g.

Calories based on 1 portion of ingredients.

Breakfast Quinoa

Do you love hot breakfast cereal but you're tired of the same old thing. This hot cereal is a great alternative to what you're used to. With vanilla flavor and a hint of apple, it's sure to wake your taste buds up. Try this easy to make recipe the next time you want a hot, filling breakfast.

Ingredients:

- 1 cup washed quinoa
- 2 cups unsweetened apple juice
- 2 cups unsweetened almond milk or fat free milk
- 2 teaspoons ground cinnamon
- 1 ½ cups raisin
- 2 teaspoons vanilla extract

Instructions:

Make sure that all cooking surfaces and utensils are clean before staring.

To begin, thoroughly rinse the quinoa. In a 12-quart pan, bring quinoa to a boil with apple juice. Once at a boil, reduce heat and simmer until the apple juice is almost completely dissolved. Add milk, raisins and cinnamon and cover with a fitted lid. Simmer for 15 minutes, occasionally stirring the ingredients.

Remove from heat. The vanilla extract should now be stirred in.

*Tips and Suggestions: This recipe can be served hot or cold. Raisins can be substituted with Craisins, or eliminated for lower sugar. This serves mainly as a carb source, so eat alongside egg whites or a protein shake for a complete meal.

Cooking time (duration): 40 minutes

Serves: 6 Nutritional Values: 228 Calories per serving. Total Fat: 12.2 g, Cholesterol: 0.6 mg, Sodium: 169.9 mg, Total Carbs: 28.4 g, Protein: 9.3 g

Calories based on 6 equal portions of ingredients.

Cinnamon Raisin Rice Breakfast

Oatmeal isn't the only option when you want to enjoy hot breakfast cereal. Brown rice can be used to fill you up the same way. Using this recipe, you can have something different for a change and still have a healthy breakfast. Brown rice isn't just for dinner anymore.

Ingredients:

- ½ cup brown rice
- ½ cup unsweetened almond milk or fat free milk
- ½ teaspoon cinnamon
- *1-tablespoon raisins (1/4 small 1.5 oz. box)
- 1 teaspoon sliced almonds
- 1 tablespoon Splenda or 1 packet Truvia

Instructions:

Clean all cooking utensils and work surfaces before you begin cooking.

Combine all ingredients in a medium saucepan. Cook over medium heat.

*Tips and Suggestions: This brown rice dish should have the same consistency as oatmeal when it's done. The low-fat milk in this recipe can be substituted with soymilk. *Raisins during maintenance phase only. This is a carb source, so eat alongside egg whites, lean turkey bacon or a protein shake for a complete meal.

Serves: 2   Nutritional Value: Calories per serving: 165 g; Total Fat: 4.8 g (0.4 g sat), Cholesterol: 2.5 mg, Sodium: 66.2 mg, Total Carbs: 25.4 g, Protein: 7.6 g; Fiber: 2.1 g.

Calories based on 2 equal portions of ingredients.

Simple Spiced Oatmeal

On a cold winter morning, there's nothing like a bowl of hot oatmeal. Even if you're rushing in the morning, you'll have time to make this quick and filling meal. It only takes a few minutes to start your day off with a healthy breakfast. Use this easy oatmeal recipe to get a spicy start to your day.

Ingredients:

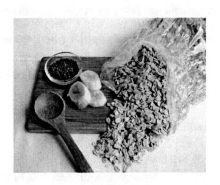

　　1 cup raw oats
　　2 cups water
　　1/8 teaspoon salt
　　1 small ripe banana, sliced
　　¼ teaspoon cinnamon
　　¼ teaspoon nutmeg
　　1 teaspoon ground flax seed
　　1 tablespoon fat free skim milk

Instructions:

Be certain that all cooking surfaces and utensils are clean prior to cooking.

In a medium saucepan, add all ingredients except the ground flax seed. Cook over medium heat until ingredients begin to simmer. Add ground flax seed and milk.

*Tips and Suggestions: Try fruits like peaches, berries or apples in place of the banana. You can also add allspice to your oatmeal. For a sweetener during maintenance phase, use a teaspoon of Splenda or Stevia or a packet of Truvia. This meal is mainly carbohydrate, so eat alongside egg whites or a protein shake to meet protein goals. Eliminate fruits for less sugar.

Cooking time (duration): 8 minutes

Serves: 2 Nutritional value per serving: 205.8 Calories; Fat: 3.7 g (0.7 g sat); Sodium: 86.9 mg; Carbohydrates: 41.6 g; Protein: 6.0 g; Fiber: 5.8g.

Calories based on 2 equal portions of ingredients.

Mini Veggie Breakfast Muffins

Veggies are making a morning salute! Most people only think of vegetables when it's time for lunch and dinner but they are a great addition to any recipe. These mini veggie bakes are ideal for a filling breakfast that will help curb your appetite throughout the day. Fun, cute and petite, they are ready to go when you are.

Ingredients:

> 1½ cups egg substitute or 6 egg whites, stirred
> 1 cup cooked broccoli
> 2 cups baby spinach, sautéed
> 2 tablespoons chopped shallots
> 1 cup cooked asparagus
> ½ cup cherry tomatoes, quartered
> ¼ cup low-fat cheese blend (any cheese you like will do)

Instructions:

Set the oven to 350 degrees to preheat.

Sauté broccoli, spinach, shallots, and asparagus in a nonstick pan, or lightly coat a pan with 1 tablespoon of olive oil. Set vegetable mixture aside in a bowl and cool to room temperature.

Quarter tomatoes so there is enough to put at least 3 pieces into each muffin.

Spray the muffin tin with olive oil spray, or use silicone muffin liners. Place about 1/8 cup of sautéed vegetable mixture in each tin of a 12-cup muffin pan. Using ¼ cup measuring scoop, add mixed egg substitute or egg whites to each tin. Sprinkle a pinch of cheese over the top and bake for 30 minutes. Muffins can be eaten immediately.

*Tips and Suggestions: Store muffins in the refrigerator or freezer after they have completely cooled. You can use any vegetable you like with this recipe, a mixture or just one. Adding some Jennie O's lean turkey bacon would enhance the flavor and protein, but only during the maintenance phase.

Cooking time (duration): 45 minutes; Serves: 6 Nutritional Value per serving: 60 Calories; Fat: 0.5 g; Cholesterol: 1.6 mg; Sodium: 163 mg; Total Carbs: 4.9 g; Protein: 8.8 g; Fiber: 1.7g.

Calories based on 6 equal portions of ingredients.

Spinach Quiche Breakfast Cupcakes

Cupcakes for breakfast are a "no-no", unless your cupcakes are filled with healthy ingredients. These breakfast cupcakes are a perfect way to incorporate more veggies into your diet. Fast and easy to make, you'll have an on-the-go breakfast in less than an hour.

Ingredients:

5 large eggs or 1¼ cups egg substitute
1 10oz. package frozen spinach
1 cup of low-fat cheddar cheese
½ teaspoon baking powder
½ teaspoon paprika
Dash salt
Dash pepper

Instructions:

Before beginning any cooking project, be sure that all of your work surfaces and cooking utensils are clean.

To prepare, set oven to 350 degrees to preheat. Take spinach out and follow the directions for thawing the spinach in the microwave by putting it in a Pyrex or microwave-safe dish with a tablespoon or two of water and thaw. Spray a cupcake pan lightly with olive oil spray, or use silicone cupcake liners (makes 12 cupcakes).

When spinach is thawed, remove as much water as possible by squeezing it with paper towels.

Beat egg substitute, baking powder, paprika, and salt and pepper in a bowl. When blended, add cheese and spinach. Thoroughly mix ingredients together. Pour equal amounts of mixture into each of the 12-cupcake wells or into each of the silicone liners, and bake for 30 minutes.

*Tips and Suggestion: This dish is great hot or cold. For more flavors, try adding lean turkey bacon or other vegetables. You can also add fresh herbs or dried herbs and other spices such as cayenne pepper or Tabasco to give these cupcakes a kick!

Cooking time (duration): 30 minutes

Serves: 6. Nutritional Values Per Serving: 69 Calories. Fat per serving: 1.4g; Cholesterol: 4.5 mg; Sodium: 301 mg; Carbohydrates: 2.9 g; Protein: 10.8 g.

Calories based on 6 equal portions of ingredients.

Beanie Breakfast Baby Cakes

Beans are taking over breakfast. Full of protein and iron, these kidney bean and rice cakes are a great way to start your day with a healthy serving of what your body needs. Quick to make and transportable, too! Here's another recipe to add to your healthy eating list.

Ingredients:

> ½ cup kidney beans, slightly mashed
> ½ cups cooked brown rice
> ¼ cup chopped onion, plus 1 tablespoon
> ½ cup chopped mushrooms
> Salt and pepper (to taste)
> 4 slices tomato
> 2 cups fresh spinach
> 1 medium egg

Instructions:

In a bowl, mash beans until they are coarse and mushy. Mix rice in. Over medium heat, sauté onions and mushrooms for about 5 minutes. Add rice and bean mixture to onions and mushrooms and season with salt and pepper to taste.

Remove from heat and gently form mixture into two cakes. Put back in the same pan and cook on each side for 5 minutes. If necessary, use 1 tablespoon of olive oil to lightly coat the pan to prevent sticking.

In the last minute, add spinach to the pan to make the leaves soft and slightly wilted. Place tomatoes and spinach on a plate, and arrange cakes on top.

Cook egg in same pan that has already been used and place on top of the cakes.

*Tips and Suggestions: For a little spice, add a dash or two of Tabasco sauce. Only cook spinach until its soft, to help retain the nutrients it contains. Feel free to add green peppers as well.

Cooking time (duration): 20 minutes

Servings: 2 Nutritional Value Per Serving: 161 Calories; Fat: 3.2 g (0.8 g sat); Cholesterol: 81.4 mg; Sodium: 357 mg; Carbohydrates: 25 g; Protein: 9.4 g; Fiber: 6.4g.

Calories based on 2 equal portions of ingredients.

CHAPTER 5

SOUPS AND SALADS

*All Nutritional Values provided in these recipes may vary according to the food brand you choose and portion sizes. Please still be diligent about reading your labels and nutritional information. What it says on the label of the product you choose always trumps general guidelines!

Soups and Salads are healthy meals that can be eaten at any time of the day, and are especially convenient for lunch time. Processed, fast food is packed full of fat and calories, and doesn't give you the nutrition you need for your middle meal of the day.

Lunch may be a rushed affair if you are working in a busy office, however this doesn't mean there are no alternatives to buying packaged meals. You can pre-make your lunch at home the night before work quickly and cheaply. Pack a healthy salad in a lunch box. It only takes 5 minutes to throw together some greens, tomatoes, a handful of healthy nuts like almonds, and some lean chicken, and not only will you be saving a few dollars, but also your waist-line. In a pinch, a pre made protein shake will save the day, so always have one ready in case of emergency!

Depending on what your carbohydrate goals are at lunch, fast alternatives for this time of the day are baked sweet potato (Don't have time for baking? You can cook these in the microwave!) a portion of beans or brown rice. You can still eat these foods at work by precooking the sweet potato at home and then heating it up in the office microwave. Here are some more helpful tips for a healthy lunch:

Avoid High-Fat Spreads - Butter and margarine are full of fat and high in calories, so if you are making your own sandwich then use sparingly or avoid altogether. As an alternative, consider using ripe avocado as a spread, it is tasty and full of vitamins and minerals. Hummus is also a fantastic alternative, full of flavor and chock full of protein and good for you vitamins, especially if you make your own.

Try A Winter Warming Soup – Soup can be a healthy and delicious lunch when prepared on your own (pre packaged soups are often laden with sugar just like other packaged foods, so read labels wisely!). Vegetable and chicken broths offer wholesome nutrition, just be sure to choose the low-sodium variety. If you have high blood pressure, soup will not be a good option for you due to the higher sodium levels. Please do not overeat soup. Portion it out as you would anything else, and be aware that the sodium levels of even a "low" sodium option can still cause you to bloat. When protein sources are added, you can have a full balanced meal in a bowl. For soups that don't contain a whole protein source, you will want to have them as a side dish. Avoid having just a bowl of canned soup or a cup-a-soup as this isn't enough to get you through the day and is loaded with sodium.

Watch The Waistline – Stick with whole foods for the most part, but when you are buying packaged products always check the label. Many lower calorie options will contain more additives and sugar to enhance flavors. Look at the calorie, fats, sugars and first ingredient on the label to make good choices. If "high fructose corn syrup" is in the ingredients, please make an alternate choice. Your best option is to make your soups at home.

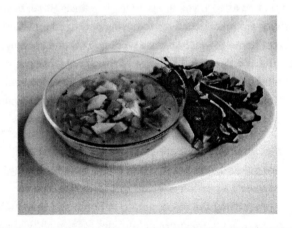

Spicy Summer Watercress and Chickpea Soup

Watercress has grown more popular over the past decade as people have realized its endless health benefits! This highly nutritious vegetable is packed full of vitamins and iron, but is also famed for its amazing anti-cancer properties. This particular recipe combines watercress with chickpeas, which are high in protein, making them an excellent meat alternative for vegetarians. For a powerful protein boost, add 1-2 cups of chopped grilled chicken or turkey breast to this recipe or eat it as a side dish with the complete protein source of your choice.

Ingredients:

> 1 tablespoon olive oil
> 1 onion, small diced
> 2 cloves garlic, crushed
> ½ -1 teaspoon crushed, flaked chili
> 1½ cups chopped tomato
> 1½ cups canned chickpeas, drained with a few reserved to garnish
> 3 cups vegetable broth or stock, preferably low-sodium (or chicken stock/broth depending on which you have)
> 2 cups fresh watercress, rinsed
> A squeeze of lemon juice
> Freshly ground black pepper

Instructions:

Begin by heating the olive oil in a large pan. Once hot, sauté the onion for 4 minutes until soft and then add the garlic and chili. Cook for a further 30 seconds. Next add the tomatoes, chickpeas and stock, stir and bring to a boil. Then cover and leave to simmer for 10 minutes.

Transfer the mixture to a food processor, and add 1 cup of the watercress. Then blend until just smooth. Now return to the pan, add the lemon juice, and season with black pepper to taste. Serve with the reserved chickpeas and 1 cup of watercress. *Tips: The flaked chili in this recipe is optional, and the soup tastes just as delicious without it!

Cooking time (duration): 15 minutes

Serves: 4 Nutritional Value Per Serving: 174 calories; 4.9 g Fat; Sodium: 994 mg; Carbohydrates: 28 g; Protein: 5.7 g. Calories based on 4 equal portions of ingredients.

Garden Vegetable Hot and Sour Soup

This tasty, Asian soup contains exotic mushrooms and bamboo shoots. You may not be very familiar with bamboo shoots, but they are full of flavor and excellent for the digestive system and high blood pressure. Give this spicy soup a try. For a powerful protein boost, add 1-2 cups of chopped grilled chicken or turkey breast to this recipe or eat it as a side dish with the complete protein source of your choice.

Ingredients:

- ¼ cup dried porcini mushrooms
- ½ cup fresh Shiitake mushrooms
- 5 cups vegetable stock, reduced sodium
- 2 cups tinned bamboo shoots, drained and shredded
- 2 cups ready marinated tofu, cut into thin strips
- 2 small red chilies, finely chopped
- 3 tablespoons white wine vinegar
- 2 tablespoons shoyu (low sodium soy sauce)
- 1 tablespoon corn flour
- 4 tablespoons water
- 2 teaspoon toasted sesame oil
- 2 spring onions, shredded

Instructions:

To prepare for cooking, first soak the dried porcini in hot water for 15 minutes. Once soaked, drain the liquid through kitchen paper and keep the liquid for later. Rinse and slice the porcini.

Now you'll need to prepare the shiitake mushrooms by removing the stalks (you do not need them in the recipe) and slicing the remaining mushrooms.

In a large saucepan add the porcini mushroom liquid that you reserved earlier, the stock and the mushrooms. Bring to a boil and then reduce the heat so that it is simmering for 10 minutes.

Next add tofu, bamboo shoots and chili, then leave to simmer for 5 minutes. Then you can add the vinegar and shoyu.

Finally stir the corn flour together with a little water to make a paste. Add this to the soup, making sure to stir constantly until thickened. Remove from the heat, season with the sesame oil and garnish with the chopped spring onions.

*Tips: Consider adding a squeeze of lime juice. This will give the soup and extra kick, and produce an authentic Asian flavor.

Cooking time (duration): 15 minutes

Serves: 6 Nutritional Value Per Serving - 131 Calories; 9.1g Fat; Cholesterol: 0.6 mg; Sodium: 998 mg; Carbohydrates: 13.3 g; Protein: 15.7 g; Fiber: 3.4g.

Calories based on 6 equal portions of ingredients.

Vegetable, Lentil & Orange Soup

This soup is packed full of flavor but with absolutely no saturated fat. It contains red lentils, which are full of protein; together with fresh veggies and no sugar added Greek yogurt provide a perfectly balanced meal. The gentle spices and yogurt complement each other beautifully. For a powerful protein boost, add 1-2 cups of chopped grilled chicken or turkey breast to this recipe or eat it as a side dish with the complete protein source of your choice.

Ingredients:

1 teaspoon cumin seeds
2 teaspoons coriander seeds
1 onion chopped
2 cups carrots diced
2/3 cup red lentils
1¼ cup orange juice (or substitute 2 teaspoon grated orange peel and increase amount of vegetable broth by 1 cup to maintain the same consistency during transformation phase)
2 tablespoons "No Sugar Added" Greek yogurt
Fresh chopped coriander to garnish
Pinch paprika to garnish
2½ cups vegetable stock

Instructions:

To begin, crush the seeds in a pestle and mortar. Pan-toast (dry, do not add oil or water) the seeds for approximately 2 minutes until lightly browned. Watch them carefully so they don't burn.

Next, add the onion, lentils, carrots, orange juice, stock and seasoning to the pan, and bring to a boil. Cover, turn down the heat slightly and simmer until the lentils have softened, which should take about 30 minutes.

Place the mixture into a food processor and blend until it is smooth. Then return the soup to the pan and gently heat. Finally, serve the soup in individual bowls, with a small amount of the yogurt as a topping and some coriander and paprika to garnish.

*Tips: If you don't own a pestle and mortar then place the seeds in a small plastic bag and crush using a rolling pin. You could also use pre-ground cumin. Using the seeds with the pestle and mortar just provides a more fresh, vibrant flavor. Also, during the transformation phase, this recipe could be used by exchanging the orange juice (sugar content) with orange extract or even grated orange zest, and increasing the vegetable broth content to maintain the desired consistency. The result will be less sweet, but will still have great flavor.

Cooking time (duration): 35 minutes

Serves: 4 Nutritional Value per Serving - 126 Calories; 0.8g Fat (0g sat fat); Cholesterol: 0.0 mg; Sodium: 639 mg; Carbohydrates: 25.2 g; Protein: 5.9 g.

Calories based on 4 equal portions of ingredients.

Zesty Zucchini and Pea Summer Soup

Don't have the time to cook a soup from scratch? Well this soup only takes 15 minutes to make so now there's no excuse! This recipe contains zucchini, a summer vegetable full of vitamin A and C and fiber. For a powerful protein boost, add 1-2 cups of chopped grilled chicken or turkey breast to this recipe or eat it as a side dish with the complete protein source of your choice.

Ingredients:

- 1 teaspoon of olive oil
- 1 Bunch Spring onions, chopped
- 3 zucchinis, chopped
- 1 ½ cups fresh or frozen peas
- 3 ¾ cups hot vegetable stock
- 1 cup trimmed watercress
- 1 Handful of mint
- 2 tablespoons "No Sugar Added" Greek yogurt, plus extra for serving

Instructions:

First of all, heat the pan for a minute and then add the olive oil. Next, add the spring onions and zucchinis and stir. Allow to cook for 3 minutes. Add the peas and stock and bring to a boil. Cover and simmer for another 4 minutes and then remove from the heat. Stir in the watercress and mint and wait until they have just wilted.

Blend in a food processor in two batches. Add the Greek yogurt with the second batch. Then return the soup to the pan, and add seasoning to taste. Serve drizzled with extra yogurt.

*Tips: This soup tastes equally delicious hot or cold. On a hot summer day, it is best served chilled as a low fat tasty lunch.

Cooking time (duration): 10 minutes

Serves: 4 Nutritional Value per Serving - 92 Calories; 0.3 g Fat (0.1 g sat fat); Cholesterol: 0.0 mg; Sodium: 955 mg; Carbohydrates: 17.6 g; Protein: 5.3 g; Fiber: 4.5 g.

Calories based on 4 equal portions of ingredients.

Sea Food & Fennel Soup

This luxurious seafood bisque is perfect for a dinner party or formal occasion. Despite being a rich, flavorsome dish it is surprisingly low in calories. The soup contains fennel, which is rich in vitamins and excellent for digestive health. You will find the anise flavor of the fennel also compliments the shrimp perfectly.

Ingredients:

   3 cups raw shrimp, cleaned.
   4 tablespoons olive oil
   1 large onion, chopped
   1 large fennel bulb, chopped
   2 carrots, chopped
   ½ cup dry white wine
   2 cups canned, chopped tomatoes
   4 ¼ cups fish stock
   2 generous pinches paprika

Instructions:

Begin by cleaning and deveining shrimp. Boil shrimp until cooked (just a few minutes) and remove from the heat. In a deep sauté pan or Dutch oven, add the onion, carrots and fennel and cook for about 10 minutes until the vegetables have softened slightly. Pour in the white wine and simmer for about 1 minute until the alcohol has evaporated. Now add the tomatoes, stock and paprika. Cover and simmer for 30 minutes. While the soup is cooking, chop the shrimp.

Once the soup has been simmering for 30 minutes, take it off the heat. Blend the soup as smoothly as possible using an immersion blender, or by putting it into a food processor. Drain the soup through a sieve or fine mesh colander into a bowl to remove any large pieces of vegetable. Press the mixture through the sieve to get out the entire flavor.

Return to a clean pan, add the shrimp and cook for 10 minutes. Blend again until smooth if desired, or leave as is for a chunkier consistency and to add a texture.

*Tips: This is quite a rich dish, and a small bowl is probably enough to satisfy. This is an excellent soup to chill a day ahead of serving and can be frozen for up to a month. Flavors will be richer a day or two later. You could garnish by setting aside a few of the shrimp and sautéing them in 1 teaspoon or 2 of olive oil and placing one or two on the top of each soup.

Cooking time (duration): 55 minutes

Serves: 8 Nutritional Value per Serving - 201 Calories; 8.5g Fat (1.2g sat fat); Cholesterol: 5.4 mg; Sodium: 4.3 mg; Carbs: 10.7 g; Protein: 19.8 g.

Calories based on 8 equal portions of ingredients.

Italian Creamed Bean Soup

This recipe is a healthy, easy way to enjoy the tastes of Italian bean soup without spending hours in the kitchen. For a powerful protein boost, add 1-2 cups of chopped grilled chicken or turkey breast to this recipe or eat it as a side dish with the complete protein source of your choice.

Ingredients:

- 1 tablespoon olive oil
- 1 onion, chopped
- 1 stalk celery, chopped
- 1 clove garlic, chopped
- 2 (16oz) cans white kidney beans, rinsed and drained
- 1 (14oz) can low-sodium, fat-free chicken broth
- ¼ teaspoon ground black pepper
- 1/8 teaspoon dried thyme
- 2 cups water
- 1 bunch fresh spinach, rinsed and thinly sliced
- 1 tablespoon lemon juice

Instructions:

Before you begin cooking, be sure that all of your work surfaces and cooking utensils are clean and ready to be used.

Heat deep saucepan for about 30 seconds then add olive oil. Add onion and celery to saucepan until tender. Mix in garlic and cook half a minute. Stir beans, chicken broth, pepper, thyme and water into the vegetables. Allow mixture to come to a boil, reduce heat and simmer for approximately 15 minutes.

Remove 2 cups of beans and veggies with a slotted spoon and set aside in a bowl. Blend the remaining soup with an immersion blender, or in a regular blender in batches, until smooth. Return mixture to the saucepan and add back in the reserved 2 cups of beans and veggies.

Heat ingredients again, bringing to a boil. Be sure to stir occasionally. Add spinach to the soup and cook until wilted. Stir in lemon juice and immediately remove from heat.

*Tips and Suggestions: Serve this soup with grated low-fat cheese on top, but only during maintenance phase. It's important when removing 2 cups to set aside that there is as little liquid as possible removed with it. For more flavors, add your favorite Italian spices.

Cooking time (duration): 50 minutes

Serves: 6 Nutritional Values: 247 Calories per serving; Cholesterol: 1.3 mg; Sodium: 303 mg; Carbohydrates: 42 g; Protein: 15 g; Fiber: 10 g.

Calories based on 6 equal portions of ingredients.

Spiced Veggie Asian Soup

The Orient is infamous for spice, so it would only be right that this soup follows suit. Full of hearty vegetables and heat. For a powerful protein boost, add 1-2 cups of chopped, grilled chicken or turkey breast to this recipe or eat it as a side dish with the complete protein source of your choice..

Ingredients:

   6 cups fat-free vegetable broth
   2 cups bok Choy, chopped
   2 cups Chinese cabbage, chopped
   ¼ cup ginger, thinly sliced and julienned
   4 oyster mushrooms, thinly sliced
   2 cups scallions
   1 (8oz) can sliced water chestnuts, drained
   1 red pepper cut in half, halves cut into 3 slices the long way and then each section thinly sliced cross-wise.
   3 cloves garlic, minced
   ¼ teaspoon red pepper flakes
   2 cups snow peas
   1-cup fresh bean sprouts
   2 tablespoons lite (or reduced sodium) soy sauce

½ cup fresh cilantro, chopped

Instructions:

Clean all work surfaces and cooking utensils before you begin cooking. Put chicken broth in a big saucepan or Dutch oven to heat up.

Put all ingredients except the snow peas and bean sprouts into a large, cold pot. Add heated broth. Bring the vegetables and broth to a boil. Reduce heat and simmer for approximately 5 minutes.

Add the snow peas and bean sprouts, and cook for an additional 5 minutes. Soy sauce and cilantro can now be added in. Allow to cook for about another 3 minutes. Remove from heat. Serve hot.

*Tips and Suggestions: This soup is spicy. If you want, eliminate the red pepper flakes from the recipe.

Cooking time (duration): 35 minutes

Serves: 10 Nutritional Value: 47 calories per serving. Cholesterol: 5.4 mg; Sodium: 483 mg; Carbohydrates: 9 g; Protein: 2.5 g; Fiber: 2.0g.

Calories based on 10 equal portions of ingredients.

S.O.B. Black Bean Soup

Recipes that represent food from South of the Border are known for their heat. Fresh jalapenos are the fire starter in this black bean soup recipe. Healthy and full of flavor, this is a great variation on this classic soup that is super easy to make. *This recipe requires preparing the beans the night before serving. For a powerful protein boost, add 1-2 cups of chopped grilled chicken or turkey breast to this recipe or eat it as a side dish with the complete protein source of your choice.

Ingredients:

2 tablespoons olive oil
1 medium red onion, finely chopped
2 jalapeno peppers, chopped
3 cloves garlic, minced
1 tablespoon ground cumin
2 cups dry black beans
2 cups fat-free vegetable stock
¼ cup cilantro, finely chopped
1/3 teaspoon kosher salt

Instructions:

Clean all work surfaces and cooking utensils prior to using them.

**The night before, rinse black beans until they're clean, place in a bowl and cover with water. Allow beans to soak in the refrigerator overnight.

To make soup:

Drain beans, put in a pot and cover with cold water. Cook beans until tender. When beans are almost finished cooking, add salt.

As beans are cooking, sauté in a Dutch oven or larger, deep saucepan, onions, jalapenos, garlic and cumin in olive oil until onions are slightly tender. When the beans are fully cooked, add the beans (without their cooking liquid) and stock to the sautéed vegetable mixture. Thoroughly stir. Reduce heat and simmer for 15 minutes. Add cilantro and salt and pepper to taste.

*Tips and Suggestions: Serve with whole-wheat tortilla chips (during maintenance phase) or topped with low-fat plain yogurt or sour cream. You can also add brown rice to this soup as well.

Cooking time with prepared black beans: 40 minutes

Serves: 4 Nutritional Value: 205 Calories per serving. Cholesterol: 0 mg; Sodium: 344 mg; Carbohydrates: 27.4 g; Protein: 8.3 g; Fiber: 8.2 g.

Calories based on 4 equal portions of ingredients.

Chicken-Veggie Chunky Soup

Chicken soup is a classic that will always be around and tastes the best when it is homemade. Chunks of white meat and vegetables fill this recipe with texture and flavor that you won't believe. Instead of settling for store bought soup, use this quick and easy recipe and enjoy the tastes of classic, homemade soup.

Ingredients:

    1 tablespoon canola oil
    1 boneless, skinless chicken breast, diced
    ½ cup green bell pepper, chopped
    ½ cup thinly sliced celery

2 green onions, sliced
2 cans (14oz ea) fat-free reduced sodium chicken broth
1-cup water
½ cup sliced carrots
1 tablespoon dried dill
1 tablespoon parsley, finely chopped
¼ teaspoon dried thyme
1/8-teaspoon black pepper
Juice of half a lemon

Instructions:

Clean all work surfaces and cooking utensils before you begin cooking.

In a large saucepan, heat oil. Sauté diced chicken until cooked all the way through. Put bell peppers, onions and celery in the pan with chicken and cook until they're tender.

When veggies are tender, add remaining ingredients and simmer until carrots are tender. Taste for seasoning before serving. May need additional dash of salt and pepper or even Italian seasoning.

Tips and Suggestions: Add any vegetables you like to this recipe. Serve hot. You could also add ½ to ¾ cup of wild brown rice to make a thicker, heartier soup.

Cooking time (duration): approximately 30 minutes.

Serves: 4 Nutritional Value: 126 Calories per serving. Carbohydrates: 6.2 g; Fat: 4.3 g (0.5 g sat fat); Protein: 15.1 g.

Calories based on 4 equal portions of ingredients.

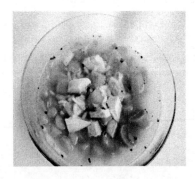

Savory Turkey and Sweet Potato Soup

Turkey and sweet potatoes are not only for Thanksgiving. This recipe combines two of your favorite holiday foods to create an everyday soup. Hearty and flavorful, this recipe is a great way to satisfy. Put a spin on your holiday favorite and have it any time you like.

Ingredients:

    4 cups low sodium chicken broth
    1 pound boneless, skinless turkey breast cut in ¾" pieces
    1 onion, chopped fine
    1 sweet potato, peeled and cubed
    1 teaspoon dried sage
    ¼ teaspoon salt
    1 cup fresh peas
    ½ teaspoon ground black pepper
    2 cups escarole, stems removed

Instructions:

Be sure to clean all cooking utensils and work surfaces before you begin cooking.

Put broth, turkey, onion, salt, sage and sweet potato in a saucepan. Boil over high heat. Once boiling, cover, reduce heat and simmer. Occasionally stir the soup and cook for about 20 minutes.

Put in peas and pepper and continue to simmer for 5 more minutes. Add escarole and cook until escarole is wilted. Serve hot.

Tips and Suggestions: Only cook escarole until it's wilted, this should take about a minute. If escarole is unavailable, use spinach or kale. Both substitutions are an excellent source of vitamins and protein.

Cooking time (duration): 45 minutes

Serves: 4 Nutritional Value: 132 Calories per serving. Cholesterol: 23 mg; Carbohydrates: 20.3 g; Protein: 11.6 g; Fiber: 4.8 g; Fat: 0.7 g (0.1 g sat fat).

Calories based on 4 equal portions of ingredients.

Auntie's Autumn Apple & Butternut Squash

As the temperatures begin to drop, you will be happy to wrap your hands around a bowl of this delicious soup side dish. This dish is a carb source, so it would not be eaten alone, but alongside your lean protein of choice. The pine nuts serve as your fat source in this meal.

Ingredients:

>   1 tablespoon olive oil or olive oil cooking spray
>   2 lbs. butternut squash (halved and seeded)
>   ¾ lb. Granny Smith apples (peeled, cored, and cut into eighths)
>   *Dice some apples for garnish
>   2 onions (cut in wedges)
>   2¾ cup shiitake mushroom caps (quartered)
>   3 cups low-sodium chicken broth
>   ¼ c finely grated Parmesan cheese
>   2 garlic cloves (finely chopped)
>   2 tablespoons pine nuts (toasted)

Instructions:

Preheat oven to 400°. Use olive oil cooking spray to coat a 9 x 13-inch baking dish. Put squash on half of pan, cut side down. Place apples, onions, and mushrooms in 1 layer on other half of pan. Roast for 45 minutes or until tender. Make sure to use middle rack in the oven for even cooking.

Remove pan from oven and turn squash cut side up to cool. After squash is cool enough to handle, remove skin from squash and put in a food processor in batches to puree. Add broth, Parmesan cheese, garlic, half of the onions and apples, and three-quarters of the mushrooms until smooth and silky in consistency.

Pour the puree into a large saucepan. Next, add the rest of the roasted apples and onions to the pan with 1 cup of water until it is your desired thickness. Bring mixture to a simmer. Remove from heat and serve. Garnish with apples, mushrooms and/or pine nuts. *This recipe would be best during maintenance phase due to the natural sugar content of the butternut squash and apples; however, if you do choose to make it during the transformation phase, limit the quantity and refrain from adding the pine nuts due to their fat content.

Total cook time: 50 minutes

Servings: 5 Nutritional Value: 243 calories per serving. Cholesterol 7 mg; Sodium: 690 mg; Carbohydrates: 44.2 g; Fiber: 9.6 g; Protein 6.4 g; Fat: 7.4 g (1.6 g sat fat).

Calories based on 5 equal portions of ingredients.

*Note: This soup can be stored in an airtight container in your freezer for up to 3 months.

Healthy Rainbow Salad

No matter what phase of life or weight loss you are in, this salad is a perfectly balanced lunch. It contains bright, colorful vegetables that are full of essential vitamins and minerals. It also has a helping of quinoa, a good source of protein and particularly beneficial for cardiovascular health.

Ingredients:

> 3 medium raw beets, unpeeled
> 6 tomatoes, halved lengthways
> 8 tablespoons extra virgin light olive oil
> 1 small butternut squash, peeled, seeds removed and chopped into cubes
> 1 head of broccoli
> 2 cups fresh peas, or ¾ cup frozen peas
> 3 tablespoons quinoa
> 2 cloves garlic, crushed
> 2 ½ cups chestnut mushrooms, or any small brown mushroom
> 2 tablespoons lemon juice
> 1½ cups red cabbage, finely shredded
> 3 tablespoons toasted mixed seeds such as sunflower or sesame
> 1 Small handful alfalfa sprouts (or a mix of broccoli/alfalfa sprouts)

Instructions:

Preheat the oven to 375 degrees. You will need 3 shelves in the oven to cook all the ingredients at the same time, or just combine the beets and tomatoes.

Place two of the beets on a small roasting tray. Sprinkle them with salt and 1 teaspoon of olive oil. Cover with foil and roast for approximately 1 to 1 ½ hours. Place the tomatoes cut-side up on another baking tray and drizzle with 2 tablespoons of olive oil. Bake them for about an hour on the lowest oven rack. Finally, put the cubed butternut squash on a baking tray and drizzle them with a small amount of olive oil and pepper. Roast in the oven on the middle rack for 45 minutes.

While those veggies are roasting, prepare the other ingredients. Bring a saucepan of water to boil and blanch the broccoli florets with the peas for a few minutes. They should still have a vibrant green color when you take them out. Drain and rinse them in cold water to cool.

Thoroughly rinse the quinoa first, and pour into another pan of water (you can use the pan of water left over from the broccoli for convenience). Simmer for 15 minutes.

Heat a pan with 1 tablespoon of olive oil and lightly sauté the garlic followed immediately by the mushrooms. Season with pepper and lemon juice and remove them from the pan after 4 minutes.

Put the shredded cabbage in a bowl. Peel and grate the remaining raw beet and stir into the cabbage. Once the roasted vegetables are cooked, allow them to cool, peeling the beets while they are still warm and then cut into wedges.

Finally, layer the vegetables in a large glass serving bowl, starting with the quinoa on the bottom, followed by the cabbage and beets, then the broccoli and peas, squash, tomatoes, mushrooms and toasted seeds.

*Tips: Simply add protein such as grilled salmon or chicken to the dish to make a complete meal.

Cooking time (duration): 1 hour 30 minutes

Serves: 6 Nutritional Value Per Serving - 277 Calories; Fat: 18.5 g (2.5 g sat fat); Cholesterol 0 mg; Sodium 40 mg; Carbohydrates 26g; Fiber: 7.2g; Protein 6.7 g.

Calories based on 6 equal portions of ingredients.

Egg and Spinach Salad

Spinach and egg are often put together in recipes because their tastes are wonderfully complimentary. This salad is great if you don't have much time, as it only takes 10 minutes to make and uses only a few ingredients that we usually have in our cupboards. The calories are reduced because six of the egg yolks have been removed (this is the part of the egg that contains the bulk of the calories).

Ingredients:

    8 large eggs
    6 cups baby spinach
    ¼ cup canned beets, rinsed and sliced
    1 cup carrots, shredded
    1 tomato chopped
    *2 tablespoons chopped pecans, toasted
    **2 tablespoons olive oil

Instructions:

Place eggs in a saucepan of water. Bring to a simmer on medium to high heat. Then reduce the heat and cook at a low simmer for about 10 minutes. Essentially you are making hard or soft boiled eggs, so only simmer them until they will be your preferred consistency on the inside.

Once cooked, drain the hot water and run cold water over the eggs until they have cooled down and you can handle them. De-shell the eggs, discarding 6 of the yolks (or save them for another recipe), and roughly chop the rest of the yolks and whites.

Toss spinach and 2 tablespoons of olive oil in a large bowl. Divide the spinach between two plates and top with the remaining ingredients.

*Tips: To toast the pecans, sauté them in a dry pan over medium heat, stirring often. They are ready when lightly browned, which should take 3 to 4 minutes. *During maintenance phase, omit the pecans, or substitute almonds instead.

**To reduce calories and fat, omit the olive oil and substitute a fat free Italian dressing.

Cooking time (duration): 10 minutes

Serves: 2 Nutritional Value Per Serving: 364 Calories; 25 g Fat (4.2 g sat fat); Cholesterol: 245 mg; Sodium: 404 mg; Carbohydrates: 16.5 g; Fiber: 5.6 g; Protein: 21.7 g.

Calories based on 2 equal portions of ingredients.

Chickpea and Red Pepper Salad with Avocado Mustard Dressing

Avocado is a healthy source of "good fat" and helps to lower blood pressure and cholesterol. This is a gorgeous summer salad, which tastes perfect for lunch on a hot summer day.

Ingredients:

½ cup watercress, large stalks removed
½ cup of black olives
½ cup baby leaf spinach
1 large carrot, coarsely grated
1½ cups cherry tomatoes, halved
1 small red pepper, deseeded and thinly sliced
1 cup canned chickpeas or dried chickpeas, cooked and drained
2 tablespoons sunflower seeds, lightly toasted

For the dressing:

1 ripe avocado
1 teaspoon Dijon mustard
2 tablespoons fresh lemon juice

2 tablespoons olive oil
2 tablespoons warm water

Instructions:

Toss the watercress, spinach leaves and carrot together, dividing between four plates. Place the halved cherry tomatoes, olives and peppers on the leaves and scatter the chickpeas and sunflower seeds over the salad.

Next, make the avocado dressing. Halve the avocado, discarding the stone. Now scoop out the avocado flesh and pulse it in a food processor, adding mustard and lemon juice. Puree until smooth, and gradually add the oil and 2 tablespoons of warm water until a nice consistency is achieved. Drizzle the dressing over the salad and serve. Season the salad with salt and pepper to taste.

*Tips: To make this a more complete meal and increase protein intake, choose an appropriately sized serving of grilled chicken or fish.

Cooking time (duration): 10 minutes

Serves: 4 Nutritional Value Per Serving (includes dressing): - 287 Calories; Fat: 18 g (2.5 g sat fat); Cholesterol: 0 mg; Sodium: 388 mg; Carbohydrates: 28 g; Fiber: 8.5 g; Protein: 6.4 g.

Calories based on 4 equal portions of ingredients.

Apple and Walnut Winter Salad

This seasonal, crisp walnut salad is perfect for refreshing your palate.

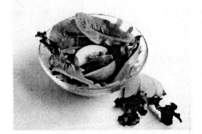

Ingredients:

1 cup salad leaves or mixed greens
5 red and white radicchio, washed and leaves separated
1 red apple, cored and thinly sliced
1/2 cup walnut halves, roughly chopped
2 tablespoons olive oil
1 tablespoons apple cider vinegar (like Bragg's)
2 teaspoons whole grain mustard
*1/4 cup low fat, Parmesan

Instructions:

Toss the salad leaves and chicory together in a bowl along with the apple and walnuts. Whisk together the olive oil, vinegar and mustard. Season salad to desired taste and spoon dressing over the salad evenly, toss to coat, and then sprinkle over cheese shavings to serve.

*Tips: This makes a wonderful starter at Christmas dinner or Thanksgiving. *Refrain from using cheese during your transformation phase. *Add an appropriately sized portion of leftover chicken or turkey and make this a complete meal, or have this as a side dish to your lean protein source of choice.

Serves: 4 Nutritional Value Per Serving: 219 Calories; 19 g Fat (3.1 g sat fat); Cholesterol: 4.9 mg; Sodium: 185 mg; Carbohydrates: 9.4 g; Fiber: 2.7 g; Protein: 5.4 g.

Calories based on 4 equal portions of ingredients including dressing.

Tuna and Olive Salad

This tasty, healthy recipe is full of vibrant Mediterranean colors and flavors. The main ingredient is tuna, an excellent source of omega 3 fatty acids that helps lower blood pressure and prevents both coronary heart disease and Alzheimer's.

Ingredients:

> 1 small fennel bulb (or you can substitute celery if you don't care for fennel)
> 1 medium red onion, halved
> 2 ½ cups canned cannellini (or other white beans) beans, drained and rinsed
> 2 tablespoons extra virgin olive oil
> 3 tablespoons lemon juice
> 1 tomato, chopped
> ½ cup fresh flat leaf parsley leaves, chopped
> 1½ cups canned albacore tuna in spring water, drained
> ½ cup black olives, pitted

Instructions:

Trim the base and top off the fennel. Core these and then slice the head across, as thinly as possible, into horseshoe-shaped slices. If you have a mandolin this would be easier. Slice the onion in the same way.

Put the chopped vegetables (including tomato) into a large bowl with the beans, oil, lemon juice, parsley and salt and pepper to taste. Stir together.

Next, break the drained tuna into large flakes and mix into the bean and fennel salad. Equally place the salad onto four plates and scatter with the black olives.

*Tips: It is best to buy the highest quality canned tuna labeled "tuna steak" to get nice big chunks. This recipe can be adapted for vegetarians by using grilled tofu instead of the tuna steaks.

Cooking time (duration): 15 minutes

Serves: 4 Nutritional Value Per Serving: 273 Calories; Fat: 10.4 g (1.3 g sat fat); Cholesterol: 15.6 mg; Sodium: 759 mg; Carbohydrates: 19.5 g; Fiber: 11.2 g; Protein 17.3 g.

Calories based on 4 equal portions of ingredients.

Tu-fu Salad

Tuna and tofu are two foods that are highly nutritious on their own. So, what so you think happens when you put the two together? This light salad is full of protein and is a fantastic way to meet your daily nutritional requirements.

Ingredients:

3 cups bean sprouts
1 package firm or medium tofu, cut into ½" inch cubes
2 (6oz.) cans tuna packed in water, drained
1 cup watercress, chopped
2 tomatoes, cubed
½ cup onion, chopped
4 cloves garlic, thinly sliced
¼ cup toasted sesame oil
½ cup light or reduced sodium soy sauce

Instructions:

Clean your work area and cooking utensils before you begin cooking.

In a dish, layer bean sprouts, tofu, tuna, tomatoes and watercress.

In a skillet, over medium heat, use sesame oil to brown garlic. Move garlic and oil into a bowl with the onion and soy sauce. Mix together, and pour on top of the prepared tofu and vegetable mixture.

*Tips and Suggestions: You can use ¼ cup Japanese pickled relish in this recipe as well.

Prep time (duration): 20 minutes

Serves: 8 Nutritional Value per serving: 162 Calories per serving; Fat: 11.8 (sat fat: 1.5 g); Cholesterol: 15.6 mg; Sodium: 399 mg; Carbohydrates: 6.9 g; Fiber: 2.1 g; Protein: 16.6 g.

Calories based on 8 equal servings of ingredients.

Spicy Pea Salad

Salads are delicious but sometimes it is fun to explore ones without lettuce or leafy greens. This recipe combines vegetables with black-eyed peas to create a salad full of flavor and fun. For a powerful protein punch, add 1-2 cups of chopped or shredded grilled chicken, turkey or eggs. Or eat as a side dish with the lean protein of your choice.

Ingredients:

    2 tablespoons fresh limejuice
    ¼ cup red onion, chopped
    ½ teaspoon ground cumin
    2 jalapeno peppers, finely diced
    1 stalk celery, finely chopped
    2 roasted red peppers, finely chopped
    1/4 cup cilantro, finely chopped
    2 (15oz.) cans black eyed peas, drained
    2 tablespoons extra light olive oil
    2 teaspoons fresh grated ginger
    Salt and pepper to taste

Instruction:

Mix all ingredients in a large bowl. Season with spices, toss ingredients together thoroughly and serve.

*Tips and Suggestions: Salt and pepper are very important to this dish because of the other spices that are being used. Also experiment with other seasonings you enjoy.

Cooking time (duration): 7 minutes

Serves: 6 Nutritional Value per serving: 146 Calories per serving. Fat: 4.8 g (0.7 g sat fat); Cholesterol: 0 mg; Sodium: 571 mg; Carbohydrates: 22 g; Fiber: 4.8 g; Protein: 6.6 g.

Calories based on 6 equal portions of ingredients.

No-egg Egg Salad

Eggs salad is a great option for a quick and easy dinner. But, what if you don't eat eggs? This no-egg recipe "egg salad" a dinner option for you again. Using tofu as the main ingredient, you can have a nutritious dinner without compromising your diet.

Ingredients:

 1 lb. tofu, firm
 ¼ teaspoon celery seed
 ¼ cup fresh parsley, chopped
 1/8 teaspoon ground black pepper
 1/3 cup celery, diced
 ¼ teaspoon onion powder
 ½ teaspoon sea salt
 ¼ teaspoon turmeric
 2 tablespoons pickle relish
 ¼ cup green onions, sliced
 1 ½ teaspoons lemon juice
 *3 tablespoons light or fat free mayonnaise

Ingredients:

Clean all work surfaces and utensils before cooking.

Remove any water or moisture from tofu by squeezing it dry. In a bowl, crumble tofu into small chunks. Add celery seed, parsley, black pepper and celery, and then add all spices. Place the bowl in the refrigerator and chill for at least 30 minutes.

After mixture is chilled, add relish, onions, lemon juice and mayonnaise.

*Tips and Suggestions: Serve this recipe on whole wheat bread or spelt bread once you are in the maintenance phase. *This recipe contains a dairy product and needs to be refrigerated. Also, during your transformation phase, you could try mustard instead of mayonnaise for a different taste, and less calories from fat.

Serves: 4 Nutritional Value per serving: Calories: 120 g; Fat: 10.9 g (1.6 g sat fat); Cholesterol: 3.9 mg; Sodium: 465 mg; Carbohydrates: 8.8 g; Fiber: 2.6 g; Protein: 13.1 g.

Calories based on 4 equal servings.

Low-fat and Yummy Fruit Salad

Brighten up your afternoon with color and flavor. Alter this recipe with the fruit of your choosing; add strawberries, pineapple, and melon or any other in-season medley.

Ingredients:

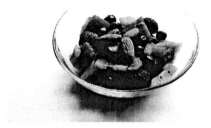

1 apple, cored and chopped
½ cup Watermelon chopped
1 kiwi, sliced
½ cup strawberries, chopped
1/2 cup blueberries
1/2 cup chopped almonds
1 (8 ounce) container "No Sugar Added" Greek Yogurt

Add Stevia or Truvia for added sweetness if desired

Instructions:

Always make sure your prepping area and work surfaces are clean. In a large bowl, combine all ingredients except yogurt. Once combined, mix in yogurt. Chill until ready to serve, or at least 30 minutes. *Because of the natural sugar content of fruit, this recipe is best used during the maintenance phase. You could also sprinkle cinnamon on top for a fresh, delightful flavor.

Prep time: 15 minutes

Serves 4 Nutritional Value per serving: Calories: 234 g; Fat: 9.6 g (0.7 g sat fat); Cholesterol: < 1mg; Sodium: 48 mg; Carbohydrates: 36 g; Fiber: 6.1 g; Protein: 6.0 g.

Calories based on 4 equal portions.

Seafood Apple Salad

Who says afternoon lunch has to be boring? Well it doesn't have to be! Try this delicious fruit and scallion salad for lunch or dinner.

Ingredients:

- 6 teaspoons extra-virgin olive oil, divided
- 1/2 cup thinly sliced shallots
- ¾ teaspoon curry powder
- 1 cup apple cider
- 1/2 teaspoon sea salt, divided
- 1 teaspoon apple cider vinegar
- 1 pound dry sea scallops, (see Shopping Tip), tough muscle removed
- 1/4 teaspoon freshly ground pepper
- 8 cups mixed salad greens
- 1 tart apple, such as Granny Smith, diced
- 1/4 cup dried cranberries
- 1/4 cup chopped almonds

Instructions:

Before you begin preparing your meals always make sure your prepping area and cooking surfaces are clean. First, heat 2 teaspoons of olive oil in a large nonstick skillet over medium heat. Add shallot and curry powder and cook, stirring, until the shallot is fork tender. Add cider and 1/4 teaspoon salt; bring to a boil and cook until reduced to 3/4 cup, about 3 minutes. Pour into a large bowl and whisk in 2 more teaspoons olive oil and the cider vinegar. Remove 1/4 cup dressing and set aside in a small bowl. Wipe out the pan.

Pat scallops dry with a paper towel and sprinkle with the remaining 1/4-teaspoon salt and pepper. Add the remaining 2 teaspoons oil to the pan and heat over medium-high. Add the scallops and cook until golden brown, 2 to 3 minutes per side. Transfer to a plate.

Add salad greens, apple, cranberries and almonds to the large bowl; toss to coat. Top with the scallops and drizzle with the reserved 1/4 cup dressing.

Cook Time: 15 minutes

Serving 4 Nutritional Value per serving: Calories: 322; Fat: 12.8 g (1.5 g sat fat); Cholesterol: 37 mg; Sodium: 202 mg; Carbohydrates: 30 g; Fiber: 4 g; Protein: 22 g.

Calories based on 4 equal portions.

Delicious Veggie Frittata

Having brunch with friends can be as simple as 1, 2, 3 with this easy to make veggie frittata. With tons of vegetables, this low calorie dish is flavorful, filling and figure friendly. With just a few simple ingredients, you can wow your guests with this low maintenance meal.

Ingredients:

    4 cups of egg substitute (i.e. egg beaters) or egg whites
1 10 oz. pkg. of frozen chopped spinach (thawed and drained dry)
1 10 oz. pkg. of frozen California mixed vegetables (contains carrots, broccoli and cauliflower), thawed
1 cup diced fresh zucchini
½ cup of a red onion, diced
1 teaspoon minced garlic
*¼ teaspoon Salt
*½ teaspoon Pepper
*Pinch of crushed red pepper flakes
*(Seasonings can be adjusted to taste)
Olive oil spray (i.e. Pam)
2 tablespoons ice water

Instructions:

Preheat oven to 350 degrees. Add 2 tablespoons of ice water to egg substitute and mix together until incorporated. Add spinach, mixed vegetables, zucchini, onion and garlic to eggs and mix slightly. Spray the olive oil in an 8-inch round cake pan and then add egg mix.

Cooking Time: Depending on your desired consistency, baking time can be from 45 minutes to an hour.

Serves: 4 Nutritional Value per serving: 198 Calories; Fat: 0.6 g (0.1 g sat fat); Cholesterol: 2.5 mg; Sodium: 676 mg; Carbohydrates: 18 g; Fiber: 5.8 g; Protein: 29 g.

Calories based on 4 equal portions.

Spicy Shrimp & Spring Greens Salad

This light and lively dish will be a hit at any party. The shrimp can be served as a crowd pleasing appetizer or added to a salad of spring greens for a first course. The blend of seasonings gives the shrimp a taste of the Caribbean with the combination of ginger, cilantro and limejuice. If you are a fan of ceviche, then you will love this salad.

Ingredients:

>   1 tablespoon of canola oil
>   2 tablespoons of fresh ginger root (peeled and minced)
>   Juice from 2 limes
>   2 cloves of garlic (finely minced)
>   1 tablespoon low-sodium or lite soy sauce
>   2 lbs. large cooked shrimp (peeled and deveined)
>   ½ cup fresh chopped cilantro
>   1 package of Spring Mix Salad Greens (4 cups)
>   ½ teaspoon honey
>   ½ teaspoon crushed red pepper flakes

Instructions:

Using a large mixing bowl, combine oil, ginger, limejuice, garlic, soy sauce, and honey and crushed red pepper flakes. Whisk together well. Add shrimp and cilantro and stir to combine. Cover with plastic wrap and put in the refrigerator up to 4 hours before placing over a bed of spring mix greens. Marinade will serve as dressing for salad.

Prep time: 10 minutes. Marinade time: 1 - 4 hours.

Serving Size: 8 Nutritional Value per serving: 140 Calories; Fat: 3.0 g (0.5 g sat fat); Cholesterol: 221 mg; Sodium: 329 mg; Carbohydrates: 2.8 g; Protein: 24.1 g.

Calories based on 8 equal portions.

CHAPTER 6
HEALTHY DINNER IDEAS

*All Nutritional Values provided in these recipes may vary according to the food brand you choose and portion sizes. Please still be diligent about reading your labels and nutritional information. What it says on the label of the product you choose always trumps general guidelines!

Dinner And Evening Meals

In the evening hours, or as you get closer to the time of day when you will be less active, you will want to eat light and be sure to include a quality protein source with your meals alongside a good healthy serving of fibrous vegetables. Most of you will want to stay away from starchy carbohydrates especially if you are looking to shed body fat, or your body easily gains fat weight. You will find a list of some of the best vegetables on page 13. For any of these recipes, if you would like to increase green veggie intake, please feel free to do so!

A good rule of thumb to follow is to make sure your last meal is at least 2-3 hours prior to going to bed, so the time of your last meal of the day will vary depending on what time you go to bed. If you eat too late and eat right before going to bed, the digestion process becomes sluggish and the enzymes find it difficult to break down food. This causes an increase in acidity, which in turn results in bloating and gas. Plan out your meals for the day accordingly. Eat your final meal of the day at a reasonable hour and brush your teeth early which will help you avoid going for a little extra "something" later in the evening!

What to Eat For Dinner

For the majority of people, dinner is the biggest meal of the day, often including a dessert. Essentially loading up on calories right before your least active time of day is not a good idea! To avoid indigestion stay away from fatty or really spicy foods at night.

Grilled Turkey Burgers and Zucchini

These simple ground turkey burgers are tasty and delicious. Eat alongside sweet potato fries as a lunch or dinner meal. For those reducing carb intake eliminate the sweet potato fries for this time of day and stick with 1-2 servings of vegetables of your choice. The recipe in this example is prepared with zucchini; however, the cooking method can be the same for any other vegetable you choose.

Ingredients:

- 1 pound of lean ground turkey (85 – 93% lean is best)
- 1-2 tsp smoked rub of choice
- 4 (1 oz.) slices of fat-free or reduced fat cheese of choice
- 1 TBSP Olive Oil
- 1-2 tsp Mrs. Dash seasonings
- 2 Small or Medium fresh Zucchini or yellow squash

Instructions:

Burgers:

Pre heat your grill to medium to high temperature. Find the leanest ground turkey available. Regular versions of turkey burger are just as high in fat as beef, so choose wisely. One pound of lean ground turkey will make 4 (4 oz) burgers, so choose the appropriate size for the amount of mouths you need to feed. Mold burgers into patty form. If you would like some additional flavor in your burgers, try mixing in a seasoning such as Mrs. Dash prior to forming patties. Once patties are formed, take the smoked rub of choice (one of our favorites is the smokehouse rub from William Sonoma) and rub ¼ - ½ tsp on the top of the burger. Place burgers on the grill and cook for 10 – 15 minutes according to how well done you would like them. Be sure to cook thoroughly and use a knife to check that the middle is cooked to your preference. If you are adding cheese, place one slice on the top of the burger about a minute before taking it off the grill.

*Tip: Serve burger on whole-wheat buns or eat them plain to reduce carb intake.

Zucchini or Yellow Squash:

Take 1-2 small to medium sized zucchini or yellow squash, slice in half and then slice each half down the middle and then into quarters. Take a large piece of tin foil and place the wedges in the center. Take a small bowl and pour in 1 TBSP Olive Oil and 1-2 tsp of Mrs. Dash seasonings. You can also add some sea salt if you would like.

Mix together and then either drizzle or brush oil lightly across the top of your vegetables. Then wrap the tin foil up into a small packet by folding the tin foil. Place your vegetables on the top rack of your grill and cook for 10 – 15 minutes.

Total Cooking time: 20 minutes.

Serving Size: 4 Nutritional Value per serving (varies depending on leanness of the turkey burger that you choose, these numbers are for 85% lean turkey meat per 4 oz portion with one slice provolone cheese and 4 oz of zucchini) If you add a bun, include those additional calories: 356 Calories; Fat: 26.8 g (6 g sat fat); Sodium: 332 mg; Carbohydrates: 3.8 g; Protein: 26.1 g.

"Just the 2 of Us" Pasta (Chicken, Spinach & Feta)

Some of the most wonderful flavors combine in this dish: Chicken, Spinach and Feta. *This recipe is best enjoyed during the maintenance phase due to the higher carbohydrate count, or could be eaten earlier when higher carb count is more acceptable.

Ingredients:

    4 oz. portion of Whole Grain Plus penne pasta
    8 oz. Grilled, chopped boneless, skinless chicken breast
    1 tablespoon Olive Oil
    ¼ cup chopped onion
    1 clove of garlic, finely minced
    ½ cup fresh mushrooms, sliced
    1½ cups chopped tomatoes
    1 cup (packed) spinach leaves
    2 oz. reduced fat feta cheese
    *Salt
    *Pepper
    *Pinch of red pepper flakes
    *(Season to taste)

Instructions:

Take pre grilled or baked chicken breast (take plain chicken breast, bake at 375 for 30 – 45 minutes) and slice into small bite size cubes. Use 8 oz or more chicken per person, depending on protein needs. You could use Turkey Breast for this recipe also.

In a large pot, boil water. Lightly salt the water to add taste to the pasta. Add pasta to boiling water and cook until pasta is al dente (or desired consistency) then drain.

While pasta is cooking, in a large skillet, heat olive oil over medium-high heat. Add onion and garlic to skillet and cook until golden brown. Add tomatoes, mushrooms spinach and pre cooked chicken, stirring frequently. Add seasonings to taste. Cook 2 more minutes to allow tomatoes to heat through and spinach to wilt. Reduce heat to medium then stir in pasta and feta cheese. Cook 1 minute more to heat thoroughly.

Total Cooking Time: 40 minutes

Serving Size: 2 Nutritional Value per serving: 477 Calories; Fat: 15.7 g (3.6 g sat fat); Cholesterol: 10 mg; Sodium: 598 mg; Carbohydrates: 48 g; Fiber: 6.6 g; Protein: 40.5 g.

Calories based on 2 equal portions.

Simple Southwestern Chicken Breast

This is a simple go-to chicken recipe for any day of the week. Just a few simple ingredients and this chicken will awaken your taste buds. This recipe is a quick "go-to" after a long day at work or just something light for lunch. Used with your choice of sides, this recipe is extremely versatile, fast and delicious.

Ingredients:

    1 tablespoon canola oil
    4 skinless/boneless chicken breast (halved)
    1 (10 oz.) can diced tomatoes with green Chile peppers
    1 (15 oz.) can kidney beans (drained)
    1 (8.75 oz.) can whole kernel corn (drained)
    1 pinch ground cumin

Instructions:

First, make sure your cooking surface is clean. Using a large skillet, heat canola oil over medium-high heat. Add chicken to skillet and brown chicken on both sides. Add tomatoes with green chili peppers, kidney beans and corn to skillet with chicken. Reduce heat to medium and let simmer for about 30 minutes or until chicken is cooked thoroughly. *Juice from chicken should run clear when cooked through. Remove from heat, add cumin and stir.

Total Cook time: 30 minutes

Servings: 4 Nutritional Values per serving: 285 Calories; Fat: 4.8 g (0.3 g sat fat); Cholesterol: 55 mg; Carbohydrates: 31.2 g; Fiber: 7.4 g; Protein: 30.5 g.

Calories based on 4 equal portions.

*Tips and Suggestions: Great with brown rice or whole-wheat tortilla.

Tricky Tofu Stir-fry

In this delectable stir-fry the tofu takes on the taste of the sauce and vegetables and no one knows the wiser. Tofu is a healthy substitute for meat and/or chicken.

Ingredients:

    1 tablespoon canola oil
    ½ medium white onion (sliced)
    2 cloves of garlic (finely chopped)
    1 tablespoon fresh ginger root (peeled and chopped)
    1 (16oz.) pkg. of extra firm tofu (drained)
    1 carrot (peeled and sliced)
    1 green bell pepper (seeded and cut into strips)
    1 (15oz.) can of baby corn (drained and cut into quarters)
    1 cup of bok Choy
    2 cups chopped fresh mushrooms
    1¼ cups bean sprouts
    ½ teaspoon crushed red pepper
    ½ cup water
    4 tablespoons rice wine vinegar
    2 tablespoons honey
    2 tablespoons lite soy sauce
    2 teaspoons cornstarch
    (*Dissolve cornstarch in 2 tablespoons water before adding to sauce)
    2 medium green onions (sliced thinly/diagonally)

Instructions:

Using a large skillet, add canola oil and place over medium-high heat. Add onion and cook for 1 minute before adding garlic and ginger. Stir together and cook for 30 seconds. Next, stir in tofu. Cook until golden brown. Once tofu has reached the desired color, add carrots, bell pepper and baby corn. Stir together then allow to cook for 2 minutes. Add bok Choy, mushrooms, bean sprouts and crushed red pepper. Combine and heat thoroughly then remove from heat. In a separate small saucepan, mix water, rice wine vinegar, honey and soy sauce. Bring combination to a simmer and cook for 2 minutes. Stir in cornstarch and water mixture then simmer until sauce thickens. Finally, pour sauce over tofu and vegetables. Garnish with thinly sliced scallions if desired.

Total Cook Time: 45 minutes

Serving Size: 4 Nutritional Value per serving: 257 Calories; Fat: 10.9g (1.3 g sat fat); Cholesterol: 0 mg; Sodium: 566 mg; Carbohydrates: 27.2 g; Fiber: 6.5g; Protein: 17.0g.

Calories based on 4 equal portions of ingredients.

Micah's Tasty Soft Shell Taco's

A great dinner choice during maintenance time! Tacos can be made in a healthy way and enjoyed by the whole family.

Ingredients:

> 1 lb lean ground turkey breast
> 2 cups shredded lettuce
> 1 cup diced tomatoes
> ½ cup fat free sour cream
> 4 tbsp taco sauce
> Low sodium taco seasoning packet
> 4 -6 mini whole wheat soft shell low carb tortilla's (La Tortilla Factory)
> 1 cup shredded low fat or no fat cheese

Instructions:

Mix lean ground turkey and taco seasoning together in a bowl. Place in skillet and cook on medium heat (could also cook in turkey burger form on the grill and just break up the burger when it is finished). Cook for 15 minutes until turkey is browned and no pink is showing. Place turkey meat into tortilla, add condiments as desired (make sure to portion properly so as to not add too many additional calories with items such as sour cream), roll taco up and enjoy!

*Tips: A lower carb option would be to take all ingredients and wrap in a large lettuce leaf instead of the whole wheat tortilla! With these tortillas, a good rule of thumb is no more than 2 for women and no more than 4 for men.

Serves 4 Tortillas: Nutritional Value per serving: Calories: 379; Fat: 8.0 g (3.5 g sat fat); Sodium: 450 mg; Carbohydrates: 27 g; Protein: 22 g.

Calories based on 4 equal portions of ingredients.

Kicking it Korean

This is another great fake out, take out meal the family will enjoy. Bulgogi, the traditional name for this barbecued beef dish is served over a bed of brown rice and lettuce for a complete meal. The kids will love the sweet taste and you will love the simplicity of this meal. A quick fix for even the pickiest eater, dinner is sure to please the entire family.

Ingredients:

1 lb. top sirloin steak, trimmed
2 tablespoons low-sodium soy sauce
1 tablespoon mirin (a sweet rice wine common in Asian cooking)
1 teaspoon fresh ginger (peeled and minced)
1 teaspoon dark sesame oil
3 cloves of garlic (minced)
1 tablespoon honey or packet of Stevia/Truvia
Olive Oil cooking spray

Instructions:

With clear plastic wrap, wrap beef and place in freezer for 1 hour or until beef is firm. Unwrap beef and cut diagonally (across the grain) into 1/16 in. thick slices. In a large plastic zip lock bag, combine beef with soy sauce, mirin, ginger, sesame oil, garlic and honey. Place marinating meat in refrigerator for 1 hour. Occasionally turn bag to marinate all sides. Spray grill lightly with oil cooking spray to prepare for beef. Take beef out of plastic bag and place on grill turning often for approx. 5 minutes or until done to your liking. Serve beef over brown rice and lettuce.

Servings: 4 Nutritional Value per serving: 264 Calories (not including rice and lettuce); Fat: 9.4 g (3.5 g sat fat); Cholesterol: 100.9 mg; Sodium: 396 mg; Carbohydrates: 7.6 g; Protein: 35.1 g.

Calories based on 4 equal portions of ingredients.

Spicy Arugula, Chicken & Goat Cheese Pizza

This maintenance time pizza is a terrific balance of savory ingredients that provide major flavor in this dish. A good combination of fats, protein and carbohydrates. Watch your portions on this one! It's tasty and easy to over do it!

Ingredients:

¼ cup coarsely chopped walnuts
8 -10 oz of pre cooked, chopped, boneless skinless chicken breast
2 teaspoons olive oil

1 cup thinly sliced red onion
1 (8-ounce) whole-wheat pizza dough crust
1 cup grape tomatoes (halved), about 30 tomatoes
1½ oz. semi-soft goat cheese (sliced) – reduced fat
¾ cup baby arugula (loosely packed)
¼ teaspoon salt
¼ teaspoon freshly ground black pepper

Instructions:

Start by preheating the oven to 450°. Place walnuts on a baking sheet and toast in the oven for 3 to 4 minutes. Walnuts should become fragrant and lightly browned. Quickly remove from oven and let cool on a plate. In a nonstick skillet, heat 1 teaspoon of olive oil over medium heat then add onion. Stir occasionally, letting onion cook for 6 minutes or until soft and golden brown. Put pizza dough on a baking sheet that has been lightly coated with cooking spray. Add toppings (walnuts, onion, tomatoes and chicken), salt and pepper then goat cheese. Bake pizza at 450 degrees for 7 minutes or until crust is lightly golden and crisp. Next, add arugula and use remaining 1 teaspoon of olive to drizzle over top. Let pizza cool before cutting. Enjoy!

Total cook time: 20 minutes

Servings: 4 Nutritional Value per serving: 321 Calories; Fat: 14.8 g (3.0 g sat fat); Cholesterol: 8.4 mg; Sodium: 402 mg; Carbohydrates: 32.4 g; Fiber: 5 g; Protein: 18.8 g.

Calories based on 4 equal portions of ingredients.

Tex-Mex Tilapia

Cooked Southwestern style, this tilapia recipe puts a spicy spin on seafood. If you like intense spice, try this easy to make tilapia recipe that's sure to make you sweat!

Ingredients:

4 tilapia fillets
4 tablespoons non-fat sour cream
1 tablespoon chili powder
1 teaspoon ground cumin
1 tablespoon paprika
½ teaspoon black pepper
½ tablespoon ground coriander

½ teaspoon cayenne pepper
½ tablespoon garlic powder
½ teaspoon crushed red pepper
½ tablespoon dried oregano
½ tablespoon dried parsley

Instructions:

Be sure to clean all of your cooking surfaces and utensils before you start cooking.

In a small bowl or container, with a tight fitting lid, mix all spices and cover.

On a flat pan, place tilapia fillets and cover tops with a layer of sour cream. Sprinkle seasoning mix over the sour cream spread. Start with just 1 tsp of the seasoning to see if it is enough, and add more if desired.

Bake fillets in the oven for 20 minutes at 375 degrees or until fillets are flaky.

*Tips and Suggestions: Save leftover spice mix by storing the container in a cool, dry place like a cabinet. Use the spice mix on other meats, like chicken and turkey.

Serves: 4 Nutritional Value per serving: 145 Calories; Fat: 3g (0.8 g sat fat); Cholesterol: 56 mg; Sodium: 92 mg; Carbohydrates: 6.6 g; Fiber: 2.2 g; Protein: 24.4 g.

Calories based on 4 equal portions of ingredients.

Salsa-topped Salmon Steaks

There are many ways to enhance the flavorful fish. This recipe uses a fruit salsa on top of salmon steaks to add a layer of flavor that is sweet and spicy. Full of color, this dish is sure to impress your dinner guests with more than taste. Put some color on your table with this easy to make dish.

Ingredients:

4 4oz. salmon steaks
1 lemon, juiced,
1 tablespoon chopped, fresh rosemary
Salt and pepper to taste
1 lemon, sliced
1/3 cup water

Salsa Ingredients:

- ¼ cup diced fresh pineapple
- ¼ cup minced onion
- 3 cloves garlic, minced
- 2 fresh jalapeno peppers, diced
- 1 tomato, diced
- ½ cup pineapple juice
- ¼ cup diced red bell pepper
- ¼ cup diced yellow bell pepper

Instructions:

Prepare to start cooking by making sure all of your cooking surfaces and utensils are clean. Turn oven to 350 degrees to preheat.

Place salmon steaks in a shallow baking dish, and brush them equally with lemon juice. Use rosemary, salt and pepper to season the fillets and pour water in the baking dish.

Place in heated oven and bake for 30-40 minutes or until salmon steaks are flaky.

While fish is baking, prepare the salsa. In a bowl, mix all of the listed ingredients and place in the refrigerator.

Serve fish with salsa on top of it.

*Tips and Suggestions: Be sure to keep salsa refrigerated. Leftover salsa can also be saved in the freezer.

Cooking time (duration): 55 minutes

Serves: 4 Nutritional Value per serving: 259 Calories; Fat: 9.6 g (1.5 g sat fat); Cholesterol: 80.5 mg; Sodium: 108 mg; Carbohydrates 14.4 g; Fiber: 2.6 g; Protein: 30.2 mg.

Calories based on 4 equal portions of ingredients.

Caribbean Jamahi-Mahi

Put a Caribbean twist on your favorite fish dinner. This Mahi-Mahi dish can be made spicy or mild, depending on how much heat you like. The next time you want to show off your cooking skills, treat your family and friends to a little taste of the tropics. They'll never know how easy it really was.

Ingredients:

12 oz. Mahi-Mahi
1 cup finely chopped coconut
2 eggs
½ cup whole-wheat flour or almond flour
Salt and Pepper to taste
2 tablespoons Jamaican Jerk Seasoning (your choice of mild or spicy)

Instructions:

Always prepare by cleaning all working surfaces and cooking utensils before you begin.

Turn oven on 350 degrees to preheat. Lightly coat a baking pan with olive or canola oil.

Cut 12 oz. of Mahi-Mahi into 3 oz. pieces. There should be 4 total.

Mix whole-wheat flour, salt and pepper in a bowl. In a separate bowl, lightly beat 2 eggs. Add Jamaican jerk seasoning to eggs and beat until seasoning is incorporated throughout.

Put chopped coconut on a plate and spread out evenly. Coat the fish in flour mixture to cover on all sides.

Next, dip the fish in the egg and jerk seasoning mix. Once the fish is wet, coat in coconut.

Bake fish on baking sheet until coconut is toasty brown and fish is flaky.

*Tips and Suggestions: Cayenne pepper can be used, to taste, in place of the jerk seasoning. If necessary, use nonstick foil to bake fish. Test flakiness of fish by using fork. Also, a salsa or salad on the side would be a perfect addition. During maintenance, 2 or 3 tbsp of finely chopped macadamia nuts would also add another element of delightful crunch.

Cooking time (duration): 25 minutes

Serves: 4 Nutritional Values per serving: 264 Calories; Fat: 10.5 g (6.7 g sat fat); Cholesterol: 173 mg; Sodium: 223 mg; Carbohydrates: 18.6 g; Fiber: 3.6 g; Protein: 25.8 g.

Calories based on 4 equal portions of ingredients.

Grilled Tilapia with Hearty Vegetable & Brown Rice Pilaf

This rice dish is great served alone for a light lunch or as a great low-calorie dinner with sensational taste. Brown rice is such a great ingredient with vegetables because it gives the right texture and blends well with the full flavors of the vegetables. When making brown rice with any meal, it is always best to use a flavored broth to cook the rice. This will make every dish burst with flavor. For those watching 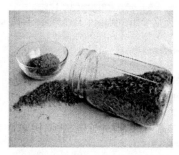 carbohydrates at night, have the tilapia and add 1-2 servings of your favorite vegetable instead of the rice!

Ingredients:

2 cup brown rice (long grain)
2 tablespoons of olive oil
4 cups of vegetable broth
2 (15 ounce) cans of black-eyed peas (drained)
1 cup sliced zucchini
1 cup sliced summer squash
¼ of a red onion (chopped)
2 teaspoons fresh parsley (chopped)
1 teaspoon fresh basil (chopped)
1 (16 ounce) can of chopped tomatoes
4 (4 - 5 oz.) Tilapia fillets
*(Use seasonings according to your taste)

Instructions:

Brown Rice and Vegetables

Using a heavy skillet (with a tightly fitting lid), heat 1 tablespoon of olive oil. Add brown rice and allow rice to toast lightly while stirring for approximately 5 minutes. Add vegetable broth to skillet, stir to incorporate, then cover tightly and cook for 45 minutes over medium heat.

In a separate pan, add remaining 1 tbsp. of olive oil and heat for a minute before adding onion, zucchini and squash until tender. Add tomatoes and black-eyed peas and mix together. Turn off heat and cover to keep warm. Add vegetables to cooked brown rice, and add fresh herbs. Mix together and add salt and pepper to taste. Keep warm on the stove until the fish is finished grilling.

Tilapia

Lightly season tilapia fillets with salt and pepper. Brush a small amount of olive oil on the grill to prevent sticking. Grill for approximately 3 to 4 minutes on each side depending on size and amount of heat. Remove from grill and enjoy with dish.

Total cooking time: 1 hour

Serving Size: 4 (1 cup rice per serving) Nutritional Value per serving: 429 Calories; Fat: 9.9 (sat fat 1.7 g); Cholesterol: 55 mg; Carbohydrates: 54 g; Fiber: 7.9 g; Protein: 33.8 g.

Calories based on 4 equal portions of ingredients.

Limon-Orange Shrimp

For seafood lovers, there is nothing like a dish centered on succulent shrimp. This simple dish uses citrus juices to put a splash of light fruit flavor on your table. Quick and easy to make, this dish is great for a simple dinner for two.

Ingredients:

    1 – 2 tbsp. olive oil
    28 large shrimp (ready to cook or you can peel and devein yourself)
    ½ lime, juiced
    ½ lemon, juiced
    1 orange, juiced
    2 dashes salt
    ¾ teaspoon black pepper
    2 tablespoons onion, chopped
    Olive oil

Instructions:

Make sure that your cooking utensils and surfaces are clean before you start to cook.

Coat a skillet with 1 or 2 tbsp. olive oil to prevent shrimp from sticking.

Heat skillet over medium heat and add all ingredients. Cook in skillet until shrimp and onions are finished cooking.

*Tips and Suggestions: Try adding lemon-pepper to this dish for a splash of citrus spice.

Cooking time (duration): 20 minutes

Serves: 2 Nutritional Values per serving: 271 Calories; Fat: 15.9 g (2.3 g saturated fat); Cholesterol: 149 mg; Sodium: 302 mg; Carbohydrates: 14.6 g; Fiber: 3.7 g; Protein: 21.2 g.

Calories based on 2 equal portions of ingredients.

Pink Citrus Chicken

Chicken breasts tend to be very dry when they cook. Using the right ingredients, you can have juicy and flavorful chicken with your meal. This recipe uses the juice of citrus fruit to boost the flavor and moisture of the chicken that the recipe calls for.

Ingredients:

    2 chicken breasts, skinless and boneless
    ½ cup pink grapefruit juice
    1 teaspoon olive oil
    ½ teaspoon ginger
    ½ teaspoon caraway seeds
    ½ teaspoon red chili pepper
    ½ teaspoon dry dill
    ½ teaspoon salt

Instructions:

Be sure that all of your cooking surfaces and utensils are clean and ready to be used.

Turn oven to 350 degrees to preheat.

In a large bowl, mix chicken breasts, grapefruit and olive oil. Be sure that the chicken is coated well. Mix the remaining dry ingredients together.

Lay chicken breast flat in a baking dish. Season the top generously with the seasoning mixture. Let marinade for 10 minutes.

Bake chicken in oven for 45 minutes or until cooked through.

*Tips and Suggestions: To add more flavors, use lemon, lime and orange juices. You may use seasonings to taste.

Cooking time (duration): 1 hour and 10 minutes

Serves: 3 (at about 4 oz of chicken each) Nutritional Values per serving: 211.5 Calories; Fat: 3.9 g (0.8 g sat fat); Cholesterol: 91 mg; Sodium: 491 mg; Fiber: 1.0 g; Protein: 37 g.

Calories based on 3 equal portions of ingredients.

Savory Sage Turkey Breast

Turkey breast is at its best when it's full of flavor that bursts. This recipe gives you a sage coated turkey breast that is so delicious you'll be upset when it's all gone. Sage is the star of the show in this easy to make, turkey breast recipe.

Ingredients:

1 tablespoon sage
1½ teaspoons seasoned salt
½ teaspoon ground black pepper
1 5 lb. turkey breast, skinless and boneless
1 cup water

Instructions:

First, you should clean all of your work surfaces and cooking utensils. Turn oven to 350 degrees to preheat. You will need a thermometer to test for doneness.

In a bowl, combine sage, seasoned salt and pepper. Coat the surface of turkey breast with seasoning mixture. Be sure to get under the skin. Cover the turkey breast with foil, loosely.

Put turkey breast in the oven for an hour. Take the turkey out, pour water into the pan and put back in the oven for 1 to 1½ hours more or until an inserted thermometer reads 170 degrees.

When done, take the turkey out and let the turkey breast stand for at least 15 minutes before slicing.

*Tips and Suggestions: Baste the turkey breast as it cooks to help retain the turkey's moisture.

Cooking time (duration): 2 hours and 40 minutes

Serves: 15 Nutritional Value per serving: 214 Calories; Fat: 5.4 g (1.8 g sat fat); Cholesterol: 98 mg; Fiber: 0.1 g; Carbohydrates: 1.9 g; Protein: 39 g.

Calories based on 15 equal portions of ingredients.

Brown Rice, Mushroom and Tofu Curry

Curry is used for so much more than flavoring meat dishes. This dish is ideal for vegetarians who enjoy the spice of curry. Quick and easy to make, this recipe is layered with texture.

Ingredients:

> ½ tablespoon olive oil
> 1 ¼ cup onion, chopped
> 8 oz. tofu
> 6 medium fresh mushrooms, sliced
> 1 teaspoon curry powder
> 1 cup precooked brown rice
> 1 tablespoon basil

Instructions:

Clean all utensils and cooking surfaces before you start cooking.

In a saucepan, cook onions in olive oil until they are translucent. This should take about 4 minutes. Add tofu and cook an additional 4 minutes, stirring while cooking. Add mushrooms to the pan and continue to cook for 2-3 minutes.

The rice and curry can now be stirred in. Mix the ingredients in the pan together thoroughly. Add water in ½ tablespoon increments if moisture is needed. Top the recipe with basil.

*Tips and Suggestions: Add vegetables of your choice to this recipe for a splash of color. This recipe is a good source of protein.

Cooking time (duration): 25 minutes

Serves: 2 Nutritional Value: 282 Calories; Fat: 14.7 g (2.2 g sat fat); Cholesterol: 0.0 mg; Sodium: 22.5 mg; Carbohydrates: 38.4 g; Protein: 23.1 g.

Calories based on 2 equal portions of ingredients.

Elk Fajita Stir-fry

Why have the same old boring fajitas? Spice your fajitas up with flavors that will make your mouth happy. Use this recipe to change your fajita game, by using game meat! You can serve over brown rice or with a wheat tortilla wrap.

Ingredients:

    1-2 tablespoons olive oil – or Olive Oil Cooking spray
    4 lbs. elk meat, in strips
    6 cloves garlic, chopped
    6 tablespoons lemon juice
    1½ tablespoons cumin
    1 tablespoon seasoned salt
    1½ teaspoons chili powder
    1 teaspoon crushed red pepper flakes
    4 cups onions, in strips
    4 cups green pepper, in strips

Instructions:

You will need a large skillet and a crock-pot for this recipe.

Lightly coat the skillet with olive oil or cooking spray to prevent sticking. When skillet has been heated over medium heat, add meat to skillet and brown thoroughly. Cook until all sides are evenly browned, but not cooked through. Brown meat in batches to ensure that all meat is thoroughly heated. When meat is cooked, place it into the crock-pot.

Use spices to season meat in crock-pot. Add water if meat is dry. Cook for 2 hours on high. Add vegetables to crock pot and cook for another hour. Stir occasionally.

*Tips and Suggestions: Leftovers can be stored in the freezer. Try Venison or other lean wild game!

Cooking time (duration): 4 hours

Serves: 15 Nutritional Value per serving: 210 Calories; Fat: 2.6 g (0.9 g sat fat); Cholesterol: 88 mg; Sodium: 544 mg; Fiber: 1.4 g; Carbohydrates: 7.5 g; Protein: 37.6 g.

Calories based on 15 equal portions of ingredients.

No-dough Chicken Eggplant Pizza

Now you can have pizza without the traditional crust and high carbs. Try this incredibly easy and filling recipe and enjoy one of your favorites again!

Ingredients:

> 1 eggplant – 3" diameter, peeled and cut into 4 thick slices
> 4 teaspoons olive oil
> ½ teaspoon salt
> 1/8 teaspoon ground black pepper
> ½ cup fresh tomatoes, finely diced
> 1 cup pre cooked, chopped boneless skinless chicken breast
> ½ cup shredded fat free mozzarella cheese (or low fat parmesan)

Instructions:

Turn oven to 425 degrees to preheat.

Grill or bake boneless, skinless chicken breast ahead of time, and chop into small cubes.

Using olive oil, lightly brush both sides of the eggplant and sprinkle with salt and pepper.

Place eggplant slices onto a baking sheet and cook in the oven until they're browned and close to tender. This should take about 7 minutes. Only turn the slices once.

Spread a tablespoon of tomatoes and ¼ cup chopped chicken over each slice and top with shredded cheese. Return pan to oven and allow cheese to melt. Serve hot.

*Tips and Suggestions: You can use pasta sauce if you like instead of the tomatoes, but be sure to find one like Classico's tomato/basil that has no more than 40 calories per half cup, and has 4 grams or less of sugar per serving. Feel free to use whatever low-fat cheeses you like when you are in maintenance.

Cooking time (duration): 17 minutes

Serves: 4 Nutritional Value per serving: 157 Calories; Fat: 5.8 g (0.7 g sat fat); Cholesterol: 2.5 mg; Sodium: 757 mg; Carbohydrates: 9.0 g; Fiber 3.1 g; Protein: 13.4 g.

Calories based on 4 equal portions of ingredients.

Baked Herbed Chicken

Ingredients:

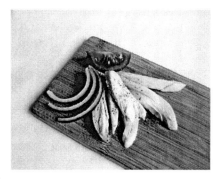

3 tablespoons olive oil
1 tablespoon minced onion
1 clove crushed garlic
1 teaspoon dried thyme
½ teaspoon dried rosemary, crushed
¼ teaspoon ground sage
¼ teaspoon dried marjoram
½ teaspoon salt
½ teaspoon ground black pepper
1/8 teaspoon hot pepper sauce
4 chicken breast halves, boneless and skinless
1 ½ tablespoons chopped fresh parsley

Instructions:

Preheat oven to 425 degrees F.

In a bowl, prepare the chicken seasoning by mixing the olive oil, onion, garlic, thyme, rosemary, sage, marjoram, salt, pepper, and hot pepper sauce in a Ziploc bag.

Add chicken breasts to a Ziploc bag with seasonings, and thoroughly coat. Store in refrigerator for at least 15 minutes or overnight, turning occasionally to ensure the chicken is coated evenly. Place the chicken in a shallow baking dish with the seasoning juice. Cover.

Roast at 425 degrees F, basting occasionally with pan drippings, for about 35 to 45 minutes. Remove to warm platter, spoon pan juices over, and sprinkle with fresh parsley.

Nutritional Information

Serves: 4 Nutritional Value per serving: Calories: 290; Fat: 12.8 g (2.1 g sat fat); Cholesterol: 103 mg; Sodium: 413 mg; Carbohydrates: 1.1 g; Fiber: 0.4 g; Protein: 41.1 g.

Calories based on 4 equal portions of ingredients.

Casseroles and Side Dishes

*All Nutritional Values provided in these recipes may vary according to the food brand you choose and portion sizes. Please still be diligent about reading your labels and nutritional information. What it says on the label of the product you choose always trumps general guidelines!

Tasty Skillet Tunarole

Tuna is for more than sandwiches. In this recipe, it is the star of the casserole. With veggies and the perfect seasonings, you'll enjoy the taste of tuna like you never have before. *Best during maintenance phase due to pasta, flour and dairy content.

Ingredients:

8 oz. whole-wheat egg noodles (e.g. Ronzoni Healthy Harvest)
1 tablespoon extra-virgin olive oil
1 medium onion, finely chopped
8 oz. mushroom, sliced
½ teaspoon salt
6 tablespoons whole wheat flour, unbleached (or almond flour)
3 cups unsweetened almond milk or fat free milk
½ teaspoon freshly ground pepper
12 oz. canned, drained chunk light tuna
1 cup peas, frozen or fresh
1 cup finely grated Parmesan Cheese
½ cup coarse Panko bread crumbs

Instructions:

Cook noodles in a pot of boiling water until they are al dente. Drain and rinse the noodles when they're done.

Preheat the broiler on your oven.

Heat a medium-sized skillet, add olive oil, and sauté mushrooms and onions with salt. Cook until onions are nicely browned. Sprinkle flour over the vegetables and integrate well.

Add milk and pepper. Stir as ingredients come to a simmer. Add peas and ½ cup of the Parmesan Cheese. Remove skillet.

Place cooked ingredients in an oven-safe dish. Cover the ingredients with breadcrumbs and remaining ½ cup of cheese. Place in oven and broil until lightly browned.

*Tips and Suggestions: If you do not have Panko, use whole wheat bread, with crusts trimmed to make homemade breadcrumbs. Tear bread and use food processor.

Cooking time (duration): 40 minutes

Serves: 8 Nutritional Value per serving: 313 Calories; Fat: 7.9 g (3.2 g sat fat); Cholesterol: 32 mg; Sodium: 455 mg; Carbohydrates: 37.9 g; Protein: 23.9 g.

Calories based on 8 equal portions of ingredients.

Chick-Veggie Casserole

Casseroles are a great way to have a whole meal in one dish. This recipe incorporates the protein of chicken with the vitamins and minerals of veggies. *Because of all the components, including pasta and cheese, reserve this recipe for maintenance. Be aware of portion sizes as casserole dishes are easy to overeat!

Ingredients:

   12 oz. poached, boneless and skinless chicken breast cubed in ½" cubes
   7 oz. whole-wheat penne pasta
   2 tablespoons olive oil
   2 tablespoons whole wheat, unbleached all-purpose flour (or almond flour)
   10 oz. low-fat milk
   1 pinch white pepper
   1 teaspoon Italian seasoning
   1 tablespoon grated low-fat Parmesan cheese
   1 yellow bell pepper, chopped
   1 orange bell pepper, chopped
   1 zucchini, chopped
   12 oz. broccoli, chopped
   1/3 cup low-fat Monterey jack cheese
   Nonstick cooking spray

Instructions:

Preheat Oven to 350 and spray 9x13 casserole dish with nonstick spray.

Chicken: To poach: Place chicken in water that covers the chicken in a saucepan with a lid. Cook over low to medium heat until chicken is cooked through. Remove the chicken from the water and cube.

Pasta: While chicken is poaching, cook pasta to al dente in a separate pot. When the pasta is about to be removed from heat, add broccoli to water and simmer. Drain.

Once you have placed the chicken in one pot, the pasta in another pot, start on the sauce. To make the sauce, put olive oil in a preheated saucepan. Once heated, stir in flour. Add milk and stir until bubbling. Lower heat and simmer for 10 minutes. Add seasoning, Parmesan cheese, peppers and zucchini. Combine well. *Reserve the Monterey jack to sprinkle over the top of the casserole.

Combine pasta mixture with chicken mixture in a bowl. Cover with sauce and stir to evenly distribute the sauce, and place in baking dish. Cover with remaining Monterey Jack cheese and tinfoil. Bake in oven for approximately half hour. Uncover and let cheese finish melting and start to bubble.

*Tips and Suggestions: Chicken can be prepared the night before. Cover and refrigerate until ready to use.

Cooking time (duration): 43 minutes

Serves: 6 Nutritional Value per serving: 298 Calories. Fat: 8.6 g (2.4 g sat fat); Cholesterol: 41 mg; Sodium: 117.4 mg; Carbohydrates: 37 g; Fiber: 6.2 g; Protein: 22.6 g.

Calories based on 6 equal portions of ingredients.

Yummy Yam Bake

Yams are a great source of healthy carbohydrates. Try this delicious recipe and feel like you're trying your yams for the first time! This recipe serves as the carb portion of your meal and is best alongside your choice of lean protein such as fish, chicken or turkey.

Ingredients:

   1¼ cup yams, diced (if you can't find yams, add 1 extra cup of sweet potatoes)
   1 cup carrots, chopped
   4 tablespoons onion, finely chopped
   ¼ cup cinnamon
   ¼ cup Splenda brown sugar or honey or agave nectar – or for less sugar choose stevia or truvia.
   3 cups Sweet potato, diced
   3 tbsp. olive oil

Instructions:

Preheat oven to 325. Place all vegetables on a baking sheet; drizzle olive oil over the vegetables. Add spices and bake.

Place the baking sheet in oven and bake until vegetables can be mashed. This can take 45 minutes or more. Once they are done, place in a bowl and mash with beaters, or eat as is.

*Tips and Suggestions: This dish can be served mashed or diced. Sweetener and cinnamon are optional. You may also want to try adding garlic or raisins to the recipe.

Cooking time (duration): 90 minutes

Serves: 10 Nutritional Value per serving: 133 Calories; Fat: 8.6 g (2.4 g sat fat); Cholesterol: 41 mg; Sodium: 117.4 mg; Carbohydrates: 37 g; Fiber: 6.2 g; Protein: 22.6 g.

Calories based on 10 equal portions of ingredients as listed.

Turnip Au 'gratin

This recipe is an alternative to potatoes au' gratin and uses turnips instead. This meal serves as a carb and fat source, and needs to be consumed alongside a protein source such as grilled chicken, fish or turkey. *During the transformation phase, you could try this without the cheese!

Ingredients:

    4 medium turnips
    2 tablespoons olive oil
    1 cup low fat shredded Swiss cheese (or low fat cheese of choice)
    ¼ teaspoon black pepper (optional)
    ¼ teaspoon allspice (optional)
    Dash salt (optional)

Instructions:

First, peel turnips and slice them into ¼" pieces. In a pan with salted water, boil turnips for approximately 5 minutes. Coat a 9" round pan with 1 tbsp of olive oil and place the turnip slices in the bottom of the pan. Drizzle the remaining 1 tbsp olive oil over the turnips and top with shredded cheese. Sprinkle turnips with pepper, salt and allspice (optional).

Bake the dish in a 400-degree oven for about 15 minutes or until the cheese has melted.

*Tips and Suggestions: Feel free to add multiple cheeses for more flavors.

Cooking time (duration): 30 minutes

Serves: 8 Nutritional Value per serving: 98 Calories. Fat: 7.3 g (2.9 g sat fat); Cholesterol: 12.4 mg; Sodium: 76 mg; Carbohydrates: 4.5 g; Fiber: 1.1 g; Protein: 4.4 g.

Calories based on 8 equal portions of ingredients.

Not "Fried" White Potatoes

Fried foods may be one of your comfort foods that will be hard to give up when you are beginning a healthier eating lifestyle. This recipe gives you the same crispiness that you have with your fries without all of the "bad" fats and calories. So, the next time you want some fries, oven "fry" them. This recipe serves as a carb source and would need to be eaten alongside a protein such as grilled chicken, turkey or fish.

Ingredients:

   2 tsp. olive oil
   2 white, yellow or red (or mix a few!) medium to large potatoes
   1 egg white (or ¼ cup of egg substitute)
   1 teaspoon cayenne powder
   ½ tsp salt
   ½ tsp pepper

Instructions:

Turn oven on to 450 degrees to preheat.

After washing potatoes, cut into 8 long wedges and dry them.

Mix egg white, seasoning, salt and pepper in a bowl. Put wedges into the mixture and coat them well. Place wedges on baking sheet in a single layer after shaking off excess egg white. Drizzle olive oil over the potatoes.

Bake potatoes for approximately 30 minutes. Turn potatoes twice while baking and cook until golden. Potatoes should be crispy on the outside.

When potatoes are done, remove and sprinkle with more seasoning to taste. Serve immediately.

*Tips and Suggestions: Any type of chili-style powder can be used for this recipe. You can also use paprika for color, or even try smoked paprika for a smoky flavor!

Cooking time (duration): 35 minutes

Serves: 4 Nutritional Information per serving: 172 Calories; Fat: 2.5 g (0.4 g sat fat); Cholesterol: 0.2 mg; Sodium: 330 mg; Carbohydrates: 33 g; Fiber: 4.3 g; Protein: 5.3 g.

Calories based on 4 equal portions of ingredients.

Sweet Baby Carrots

This recipe will dress your carrots up so they not only look and smell great; they taste great too. Lightly coated with cinnamon, carrots have never been so pretty and fragrant! This meal would count as your carbohydrate portion of your meal, and would be consumed alongside a lean protein source such as chicken, fish or turkey.

Ingredients:

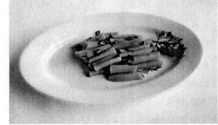

    2 cups baby carrots
    1 packet Truvia or Splenda
    brown sugar
    1 teaspoon cinnamon
    1 teaspoon olive oil

Instructions:

Clean all utensils and surfaces prior to cooking.

In water, boil baby carrots to the tenderness that you desire. Drain water and add olive oil, sweetener and cinnamon to pan and coat baby carrots well.

*Tips and Suggestions: Honey can be used in place of the other sweeteners, or omit altogether. The carrots will still taste delicious.

Cooking time (duration): 15 minutes

Serves: 2 Nutritional Value per serving: 59 Calories; Fat: 0.4 g (0.1 g sat fat); Cholesterol: 0 mg; Sodium: 89 mg; Carbohydrates: 14.5 g; Protein: 1.2 g.

CHAPTER 7
15-MINUTE MEALS

*All Nutritional Values provided in these recipes may vary according to the food brand you choose and portion sizes. Please still be diligent about reading your labels and nutritional information. What it says on the label of the product you choose always trumps general guidelines!

Chicken Fried Rice

One of the most favored Chinese dishes on a take-out menu, though at the restaurant it is not prepared in the healthiest of ways! Make this at home for a healthful option for you and your family.

Ingredients:

> 1 large egg
> 1 tablespoon water
> 2 tablespoons olive oil
> 1 cup chopped onion
> 2 cups cooked brown rice, cold
> 2 tablespoons lite soy sauce
> 1 teaspoon ground black pepper
> 1 cup cooked, chopped boneless, skinless chicken breast

Instructions:

Beat egg and water in a bowl.

Add 1 tablespoon olive oil to a skillet and warm over low heat.

Add egg mixture to the skillet and leave for 2 minutes. Do not stir the egg. When egg is cooked, remove from the skillet and cut into shredded pieces.

Now, add 1 more tablespoon olive oil to the same skillet and sauté onions until transparent. Add the following ingredients to the skillet: brown rice, soy sauce, pepper and chicken meat. Mix the ingredients thoroughly for approximately 5 minutes. Add the egg and mix well. Serve hot.

*Tips and Suggestions: If you like, use egg substitute in place of the egg.

Cooking time (duration): 15 minutes

Serves: 4 Nutritional Value per serving: 269 Calories; Fat: 9.9 g (1.8 g sat fat); Cholesterol: 79 mg; Sodium: 348 mg; Carbohydrates: 26.7 g; Fiber: 2.6 g; Protein: 18.2 g.

Calories based on 4 equal portions of ingredients.

Tasty Creamy Chicken with a Side of Brown Rice

This recipe showcases one of the many ways to use simple ingredients in little to no time and make a fantastic meal. With just 5 ingredients, this dish will become one of your favorite quick fix recipes. Done in just 15 minutes, you can have dinner on the table in no time at all giving you mounds of time to enjoy with your family. Cooking made simple and healthy!

Ingredients:

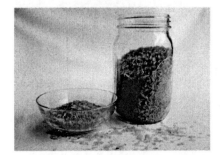

1 tablespoon olive oil
4 skinless, boneless chicken breasts
1 (10.75 oz) can Reduced Sodium "Cream of chicken with herbs" soup
½ cup unsweetened almond milk or fat free milk

Broth simmered brown rice
1 can reduced sodium chicken broth
1 cup water
2 cups brown rice

Instructions:

Heat olive oil in a skillet and cook chicken until nicely browned. Mix the can of soup and the milk in a bowl to blend smoothly, and then add them to the browned chicken in the skilled. Bring to a boil. Cover with a fitted lid and reduce heat. Cook until done. Serve over broth simmered brown rice.

*Broth Simmered Brown Rice: Bring 1 can of chicken broth and 1 cup of water to a boil. Next, add 2 cups brown rice. Cover with a tight lid and reduce heat. Allow the rice to cook until the liquid has evaporated, stirring occasionally so the rice doesn't stick to the pan. Remove from heat and fluff the rice with a fork before serving.

 *Tips and Suggestions: Use low-fat or fat-free soup, preferably reduced sodium as well. Also, you can pick whichever cream based soup you like and get a different flavor every time you make this meal. *This method of cooking the chicken is best used during maintenance.

Cooking time (duration): 15 minutes

Serves: 4 Nutritional Value per serving: 345 Calories; Fat: 7.8 g (0 g sat fat); Cholesterol: 98 mg; Sodium: 826 mg; Carbohydrates: 31.7 g; Fiber: 2.5 g; Protein: 37.8 g.

Calories based on 4 equal portions of ingredients.

Supreme Nacho Dinner

This family favorite will bring smiles to the table as the tastes of a traditional Mexican dish are served in just 15 minutes.   This recipe is fun for the whole family, but is only appropriate during maintenance and you must always be aware of the portions you are consuming!

Ingredients:

    1 lb lean ground chicken/turkey
    1 (1.12 oz) packet taco seasoning mix or 4 teaspoons
    1 (10.75 oz) can tomato soup (e.g. Healthy Request – NOT Campbell's)
    1½ cups water
    1½ cups uncooked brown rice
    1 cup Salsa (e.g. Newman's Own)
    1 cup Shredded fat-free cheddar cheese
    3 or 4 stalks of green onions, diced
    3 tbsp sliced black olives

Tortilla chips (like Trader Joe's Blue Corn Chips)

Instructions:

Cook meat in a deep skillet seasoned with taco mix. Pour off any renderings. Add rice, soup and water to the skillet and bring to a boil. Cover with a fitted lid and reduce heat; Cook for 10 minutes or until done.

Place mixture in a family-style platter and serve all the other ingredients (black olives, green onions, cheese, and black beans) in their own bowls so each guest can prepare their own nachos!

Serve with tortilla chips that are made with natural ingredients.

**Tips and suggestions: Shredded lettuce can also be used as a topping, as well as corn. For some added heat and spice, add jalapeno peppers. Also, for a bit of extra time, you can have the broiler going so each person's "nacho" plate can be heated up so the cheese can melt over the stack. Lastly, if you do not have a taco seasoning mix or packet, you can combine chili pepper, cumin, oregano, red pepper, and paprika with 1 tsp of salt and create your own mixture. Play with the portions of each to create a spice perfect for your own pallet.

Cooking time (duration): 15 minutes

Serves: 6 Nutritional Value per serving: 400 Calories; Fat: 7 g (2.1 g sat fat); Cholesterol: 56.7 mg; Carbohydrates: 27.5 g; Fiber: 3.8 g; Protein: 23.1 g.

Calories based on 4 equal portions of ingredients.

Chicken-Rice Dinner

A deliciously creamy addition to the family's cookbook, this chicken and rice dinner will became an instant hit with both family and friends. The bold taste of this meal gives the feel of a robust meal however this meal is figure friendly. This low-calorie dish is both very healthy and extremely flavorful. Broccoli gives this dish a beautiful burst of color and flavor.

Ingredients:

1 tablespoon olive oil
4 skinless, boneless chicken breasts

1 (10.75oz) can fat-free cream of chicken soup

1½ cups water

¼ teaspoon paprika

¼ teaspoon ground black pepper

2 cups uncooked instant brown rice

2 cups fresh or frozen broccoli florets

Instructions:

In a skillet, heat olive oil and cook chicken until browned.

Remove the chicken from skillet.

In the same deep skillet, bring water, soup, paprika and pepper to a boil. Add the rice and broccoli and return chicken to the pan. Season the dish with paprika and pepper. Cook until the chicken is done.

*Tips and Suggestions: To make the dish creamier, use ½ cup less rice. To reduce carb intake, eliminate the rice and just have the chicken and broccoli.

Cooking time (duration): 15 minutes

Serves: 4 Nutritional Value per serving: 400 Calories; Fat: 8.7 g (2 g sat fat); Cholesterol: 110 mg; Sodium: 725 mg; Carbohydrates: 33 g; Fiber: 4.2 g; Protein: 46 g.

Calories based on 4 equal portions of ingredients.

Super Simple Chicken and Broccoli Supper

Another variation on chicken and broccoli shows just how versatile the ingredients are, and with just a few tweaks, you have a new taste for your buds!

Ingredients:

1 package Bean thread noodles (or Glass noodles)

1 tablespoon olive oil

1 lb chicken stir-fry strips

2 cups frozen broccoli florets

¼ cup hoisin sauce

¼ cup fat-free Catalina dressing

1 tablespoon grated ginger

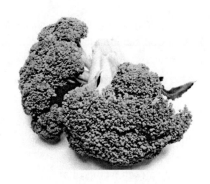

Instructions:

To prepare the bean thread noodles, soak them in water for 10 to 15 minutes, rinse and drain.

Heat olive oil on medium heat in a skillet and add chicken breast to brown.

Add florets, sauce, dressing and ginger to the skillet. Cover with a fitted lid and cook until all ingredients are thoroughly heated. During the last few minutes, add the noodles so they can be heated up. Or to reduce carbohydrates eliminate noodles.

*Tips and Suggestions: Chicken can be substituted with other lean meats. Add onions, green peppers and garlic for more flavors.

Cooking time (duration): 15 minutes

Serves: 4 Nutritional Value per serving: 201 Calories; Fat: 4.5 g (0.7 g sat fat); Cholesterol: 10.8 mg; Sodium: 470 mg; Carbohydrates: 34.1 g; Fiber: 2.9 g; Protein: 6.8 g.

Calories based on 4 equal portions of ingredients.

Quick Quesadilla

Quesadillas are always a family favorite when looking for a delicious go-to meal. Quesadillas can be made with chicken, shrimp or beef (steak), or black beans for a mouth-watering spin on the traditional cheese quesadilla. This maintenance time meal is big on taste!

Ingredients:

1 (15oz) can rinsed black beans
½ cup fresh or thawed yellow corn
½ cup low fat shredded Monterey Pepper Jack cheese (or cheese of choice)
½ cup prepared salsa, divided

4 8" whole-wheat low carb tortillas

2 teaspoons olive oil, divided

1 avocado, diced

Instructions:

In a bowl, combine cheese, beans, corn and ¼ cup salsa.

Lay tortillas flat and place ½ cup filling on each. Fold tortilla over and press to flatten

In a skillet, heat oil. Cook tortillas until golden brown on each side.

Serve with avocado and salsa.

*Tips and Suggestions: To keep warm, cover quesadillas with foil. Use fresh, prepared salsa.

Cooking time (duration): 15 minutes

Serves: 4 Nutritional Value per serving: 369 Calories; Fat: 16.4 g (3.6 g sat fat); Cholesterol: 12.5 mg; Carbohydrates: 49.4 g; Fiber: 12.7 g; Protein: 14 g.

Calories based on 4 equal portions of ingredients.

Fast Dolmas Wraps

This meatless dish has a Greek inspired taste with the mix of yogurt, feta cheese and cucumber. Fresh and light, these dolmas wraps are a great recipe for the health conscious individual looking for a low-calorie quick meal.

Ingredients:

½ cup shredded romaine lettuce

¼ cup chopped cucumber

¼ chopped tomato

¼ cup "No Sugar Added" Greek yogurt

1 tablespoon crumbled feta cheese

1/8 teaspoon garlic powder

1 whole wheat lavash*

3 prepared dolmas**

Instructions:

In a bowl, mix lettuce, tomato, cucumber, yogurt, garlic powder and feta.

Spread mixture onto lavash, top with dolmas and roll.

*Tips and Suggestions: *Lavash is thin bread that resembles a tortilla and is a great substitute for them. Nutritional value varies with size and brand. **Dolmas are grape leaves that are usually stuffed with veggies and grains. Prepared dolmas can be found in cans or jars in stores that sell Middle Eastern food products.

Cooking time (duration): 15 minutes

Serves: 1 Nutritional Value per serving: 188 Calories; Fat: 6.5 g (2.6 g sat fat); Cholesterol: 10 mg; Carbohydrates: 15.5 g; Fiber: 4.3 g; Protein: 22.2 g.

BBQ Burrito

Another favorite Mexican meal that can be made in a combination of ways in just 15 minutes or less can be both healthy and money saving. BBQ burritos are a great way to utilize leftovers with a bit of pizzazz. Using your choice of chicken, pork or lean beef, your family will enjoy this meal until the last bite.

Ingredients:

    1 (2-lb) roasted or baked boneless, skinless chicken, shredded
    3 tablespoons low sugar or sugar free barbeque sauce
    1 cup canned, rinsed black beans
    ½ cup drained canned corn
    ¼ cup fat free sour cream
    4 leaves romaine lettuce
    4 10" whole-wheat tortillas

Instructions:

Add chicken, barbeque sauce, beans, corn and sour cream to a skillet warmed over medium heat. Cook for 5 minutes.

Put a leaf of lettuce in the center of flattened tortilla and top with ¼ of the chicken mixture. Roll and slice. Do this with each tortilla.

*Tips and Suggestions: Serve tortilla warm with lime wedges. For spice add jalapeno peppers to the mixture. *Also, be very careful with the barbeque sauce as some are loaded with sugar. Look for a vinegar-based sauce that has less sugar than a brown sugar-based sauce, or the Walden Farms variety that is sugar free.

Cooking time (duration): 15 minutes

Serves: 4 Nutritional Value: 250 Calories; Fat: 4.3 g (0.6 g sat fat); Cholesterol: 30 mg; Sodium: 680 mg; Carbohydrates: 31 g; Fiber: 10.7 g; Protein: 20.4 g.

Calories based on 4 equal portions of ingredients.

Thai Style Shrimp Salad

Using the flavors of the East, this Thai dish offers great taste without loading on calories. A dish that can be used in a combination of ways, leftovers from this recipe can be used to create a Thai Shrimp over brown rice meal, or the complete salad can be added into a wheat wrap. This dish can be enjoyed over and over again.

Ingredients:

    2 tablespoons lime juice
    4 teaspoons fish sauce
    1 tablespoon olive oil
    2 teaspoons agave nectar or honey – or use stevia or truvia
    ½ teaspoon crushed red pepper
    1 lb shrimp, cooked and peeled
    1 cup sliced red, yellow and orange bell peppers
    1 cup seeded, sliced cucumber
    ¼ cup mixed herbs (cilantro, basil and mint)

Instructions:

In a bowl, whisk lime juice, fish sauce, oil, honey or stevia, crushed red pepper in a bowl. Put the shrimp, peppers and cucumber into a Ziploc bag, and pour the mixture in. Shake around to completely incorporate. Put mixture into a bowl and sprinkle the mixed herbs on top. Portion the ingredients onto 4 equal serving plates.

*Tips and Suggestions: This shrimp salad is spicy. Remove crushed red peppers from the recipe to remove the spice.

Cooking time (for the shrimp if necessary): 15 minutes

Serves: 4 Nutritional Value per serving: 173 Calories; Fat: 4.9 g (0.6 g sat fat); Cholesterol: 221 mg; Sodium: 718 mg; Carbohydrates: 7.1 g; Fiber: 1.1 g; Protein: 24.6 g.

Calories based on 4 equal portions of ingredients.

Chinese Spiced Tilapia

Taking Tilapia to a new level with a Chinese inspired seasoning will fulfill your every craving. With a subtle hint of sweet, this savory dish satisfies your taste buds. Combine this fish with a side of sautéed vegetables or flavor infused brown rice for the perfect meal. Try this dish on your friends and it will be an instant hit!

Ingredients:

- 1 tablespoon olive oil
- 1 lb tilapia fillets
- 1 teaspoon Chinese five-spice powder
- ¼ cup reduced sodium soy sauce
- 3 tablespoons honey or 1-2 packets Stevia
- 3 scallions, thinly sliced

Instructions:

Use five-spice to season both sides of tilapia fillets. In a bowl, mix soy sauce and honey.

Warm the olive oil in a skillet over medium heat. Add fish and cook until the outer edges are solid. Reduce heat and turn over. Pour soy mixture into the pan. Allow the sauce to come to a boil. Cook fish through and allow sauce to thicken a bit. Put scallions into the pan and remove from the heat. Pour sauce from pan over fish to serve.

*Tips and Suggestions: Make your own five-spice using cinnamon, star anise, Szechuan peppercorns, cloves and fennel seed.

Cooking time (duration): 15 minutes

Serves: 4 Nutritional Value per serving: Calories 156; Fat: 6.4 g (1.6 g sat fat); Cholesterol: 45.7 mg; Sodium: 618 mg; Carbohydrates: 2.2 g; Fiber: 0.8 g; Protein: 23.9 g.

Calories based on 4 equal portions of ingredients.

CHAPTER 8
SMOOTHIES

*Due to the fruits in these smoothie recipes, they are going to have a higher amount of sugars. Therefore, these are best consumed at breakfast or early in the day, and are not good alternatives for evening meals or snacks later in the day. To keep minimal sugars in the diet don't regularly consume more than one shake per day.

*All Nutritional Values provided in these recipes may vary according to the food brand you choose and portion sizes. Please still be diligent about reading your labels and nutritional information. What it says on the label of the product you choose always trumps general guidelines!

About Protein Powder

When making your shakes, an easy way to get your protein is by adding in a scoop of protein powder. However, not all protein powders are created equal! When selecting a protein powder for your shakes, please read the label and make sure that protein isolate is the first ingredient listed. Whey concentrate is a lower quality of protein and doesn't digest or absorb as effectively. Therefore, you aren't going to get the most bang for your buck if you purchase a whey protein concentrate instead of an isolate.

Casein protein is a slow-digesting, high-source protein. It feeds your muscles over a longer period of time than whey protein. The best times to use casein are in the morning and at night before you go to bed.

An optimum shake would be made with a combination of whey protein isolate and casein. This is the ideal blend for promoting the growth of lean muscle tissue. Make your shake by mixing your protein powder with water or skim milk in a blender.

For those who don't consume animal products, soy protein is a suitable alternative. Just as with whey protein, you want to find a soy product that has soy protein isolate as the main ingredient. You could also use Egg White Protein or Rice Protein Powders.

Lean, Mean and Green: Vegetables & Fruit Smoothie Recipes. Flash frozen or fresh vegetables offer an abundant amount of vitamins and proteins, and are low in calories. Here are 13 tasty drink recipes that can be added to your daily diet.

Greens such as turnip greens, collard greens, and mustard greens are high in Vitamin C and low in calories. These vegetables can be cooked, or used in salads, smoothies and juice drinks. Add protein powder to any of these recipes and increase your energy, boost your metabolism and satisfy your hunger.

*Tips: Nutritional Value of Cooked Greens

Serving Size: 1/2 cup

Calories: 25

Fat < 1 gram

Saturated Fat: 0

Cholesterol: 0

Carbohydrates: 5 grams

Protein: 2 grams

Dietary Fiber: 3 grams

Sodium: 15 mg

Vitamin A: 7,708 IU

Vitamin C: 17 mg

Calcium: 133 mg

Potassium: 110 mg

Carotenoids: 9,271 mcg

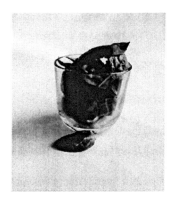

The Southern Spicy Green Smoothie

When you think about greens, most people think about home-style southern cooking and pork fat. These easy to grow vegetables are much more than just a southern tradition; they are nutritionally high in vitamins.

This tasty southern smoothie will give you the spicy flavor of the south without all the calories.

Ingredients:

  1 ½ cups Collard greens shredded into pieces
  1 cup strawberries
  1 teaspoon Cayenne pepper
  ½ jalapeno seeded
  ½ banana
  1 tablespoon apple cider vinegar
  ½ teaspoon ginger
  1 to 2 cups water
  1 scoop of Whey Protein Isolate Powder - plain
  *Ice to create desired consistency

  For an added health boost add one scoop of wheat grass or super greens!

Instructions:

Combine ingredients in a blender and add ice if needed. You can use frozen fruit (flash frozen), but fresh fruits and vegetables are always the best option.

*Tips and Suggestions: For a milder flavor, spinach can replace collard greens. Most spices such as red pepper flakes, chili powder, cayenne pepper, etc. have no calories or are very low in calories, so don't be afraid to mix and match them!

Serves: 2 Nutritional Value per serving: Calories: 182; Fat: 6.7 g; (0.4 g sat fat); Cholesterol: 21.2 mg; Sodium: 551 mg; Carbohydrates: 21.3 g; Fiber: 5.2 g; Protein: 14.9 g.

Calories based on 2 equal portions of ingredients.

Blueberry Sunrise Shake

There are days when you just don't have time to prepare much for breakfast. However, you do have time for a nutritious shake with all of the protein you need in less than 10 minutes. Don't forfeit your healthy breakfast because you have to rush. Simply take it with you.

Ingredients:

- 1 cup blueberries (or other berries)
- 1 cup unsweetened almond milk, or FF milk (or water to reduce calories)
- 1 teaspoon flax seed
- 1 teaspoon vanilla extract
- 2 oz. "No Sugar Added" Greek Yogurt
- 1 scoop of Vanilla or other preferred flavor of Whey Protein Isolate Powder

Instructions:

Add the milk or water to the blender first followed by the remaining ingredients. You can also add ice to make it more "shake-like", and pulse to the desired consistency.

*Tips and Suggestions: This recipe can be split, making two 1½ cup servings. Each serving will be half the calorie count of the whole serving size.

Prep time (duration): 15 minutes

Serves: 1 Nutritional Value per serving: Calories: 345; Fat: 2.7 g (0.9 g sat fat); Cholesterol: 35 mg; Sodium: 218 mg; Carbohydrates: 39.3 g; Fiber: 5 g; Protein: 39.2 g.

Pink Banana Protein Smoothie

Liquid breakfast can be just as fulfilling and nutritious as any other and it's faster, too. Protein smoothies are an excellent to way to get you going in the morning and boost your metabolism. Incredibly fast and easy, with delicious fruit flavor, you'll forget how healthy this smoothie is.

Ingredients:

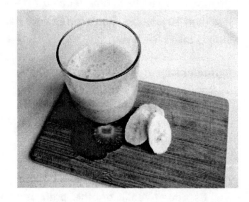

1 banana
½ cup strawberries
1 cup unsweetened almond milk
or Fat Free Milk
1 cup water
1 scoop Whey Protein Isolate
Powder – Vanilla, Strawberry or
Banana Flavors are best!
Add Stevia or Truvia if desired
*Ice

Instructions:

Add all ingredients to a blender and blend thoroughly, adding ice to create the desired consistency.

*Tips and Suggestions: This recipe can be made using a variety of fruits and vegetables. Experiment to discover new flavors. For extra sweetness, use 1 teaspoon of Stevia or honey.

Prep time (duration): 6 minutes

Serves: 2 Nutritional Value per serving: Calories 177; Fat: 1.2 g (0.6 g sat fat); Cholesterol: 17.5 g; Sodium: 95 mg; Carbohydrates: 26.1 g; Fiber: 2.5 g; Protein: 17.1 g.

Calories based on 2 equal portions of ingredients.

Virgin Bloody Mary (smoothie)

Tomatoes have proven to be a beneficial addition to your diet. Tomatoes provide antioxidants, which help prevent certain types of cancer.

Ingredients:

    2 cups tomatoes (chopped and seeded)
    ½ cup tomato juice
    ¼ cup apple juice, unsweetened
    ½ cup carrots
    ¼ cup celery
    Dash of Tabasco sauce
    2 cups of ice
    1 scoop of whey protein isolate powder – plain flavor

    For an added health boost add one scoop of wheat grass or super greens!

Instructions:

Place all ingredients in a blender and combine until smooth.

The smoothie will have a vibrant red color and fantastic taste with just the right amount of sweetness from the carrots and apple juice. Kids will love this recipe!

Serves 2 Nutritional Value per serving: Calories: 155; Fat: 1.3 g (0.4 g sat fat); Cholesterol: 15 mg; Sodium: 83 mg; Carbohydrates: 24 g; Fiber: 2.6 g; Protein: 14.2 g.

Calories based on 2 equal portions of ingredients.

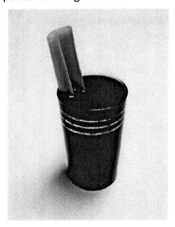

Naturally Sweet Vegetable Smoothie

As the winter season rolls in our bodies need a boost. Boost your immune system by doubling your vegetable intake. Eating fruits and vegetables are a great way to help you stay healthy and fight against colds.

Ingredients:

    1 cup apple juice, unsweetened (to reduce sugars, try this with water instead)
    1 cup of sliced apple (remove seeds)
    ¼ cup unsweetened applesauce
    ½ cup sliced carrots
    ½ cup of cucumber (peeled and sliced)
    2 cups of ice
    Dash of nutmeg or cinnamon
    Add Truvia or Stevia for sweetness if desired
    1.5 scoops of Whey Protein Isolate Powder

    For an added health boost add a scoop of wheat grass or super greens!

Instructions:

Combine all ingredients and blend until smooth. You will be amazed at the sweet and refreshing taste of this smoothie. With no added sugar or artificial sweetener, this recipe will be a family favorite.

Serves 2 Nutritional Value per serving: Calories: 221; Fat: 1.5 g (0.6 g sat fat); Cholesterol: 22.5 mg; Sodium: 72.3 mg; Carbohydrates: 34.1 g; Fiber: 3.5 g; Protein: 18.8 g.

Calories based on 2 equal portions of ingredients.

Bopping Blue Smoothie

This smoothie is so good it will make you want to dance. Kids will love the blue color and the GREAT flavor. With all natural ingredients, you will fall in love with this blend of fruits and vegetables.

Ingredients:

½ cup frozen blueberries
1 cup fresh spinach
6 oz. "No Sugar Added" Greek
yogurt
½ cup unsweetened almond milk
(or fat free milk)
1 tablespoon honey – or reduce sugars by using Truvia or Stevia

For an added health boost add a scoop of wheat grass or super greens!

Instructions:

Blueberries do not need to be thawed for this recipe. Frozen blueberries give this smoothie its texture.

Add all ingredients to a blender and blend until smooth.

Nutritional Value per serving: Calories: 233 g; Fat: 0.8 g (0.2 g sat fat); Cholesterol: 2.5 mg; Sodium: 149 mg; Carbohydrates: 39.8 g; Fiber: 2.8 g; Protein: 20.4 g.

Green Goblin Smoothie

The green color of this fantastic drink may be unappealing to adults but kids will love it. The "Green Goblin" discreetly provides kids with the nutrients and vitamins from spinach without the taste, combined with the natural sweetness of the fruits. Kids will definitely asks for seconds of this ghoulish treat!

Ingredients:

1 banana (cut in chunks)
½ apple (peeled, seeded and chopped)
1 kiwi, peeled, cored and diced
1 cup green grapes
4 oz. "No Sugar Added" Greek yogurt
1 cup fresh spinach leaves
1 scoop of Whey Protein Isolate Powder
1 cup water
Add Stevia or Truvia for sweetness if desired.
*Ice

For an added health boost add one scoop of wheat grass or super greens!

Instructions:

Prepare all fruits to be placed in blender. Combine fruits with yogurt and spinach and blend until smooth. Refrigerate at least 10 minutes, and enjoy. Serve chilled.

Serves 2 Nutritional Value per serving: Calories: 223; Fat: 1.6 g (0.6 g sat fat); Cholesterol: 15 mg; Sodium: 66 mg; Carbohydrates: 37.9 g; Fiber: 4.6 g; Protein: 18.8 g.

Calories based on 2 equal portions of ingredients.

Tropical Veggie Smoothie

Combining the melodious flavors of mango, banana and pineapple with spinach will sweep you away to the cool island breeze with one sip. The sweet and bright notes of the fruit hide the taste of the spinach while making this the best smoothie you ever tried. Both healthy and tasty, this will be a recipe you want to introduce to family and friends. It is also a great mid-day snack.

Ingredients:

　　2 cups of spinach
　　1 mango, peeled and chopped
　　1 banana, peeled and sliced
　　1 cup fresh pineapple chunks
　　1 scoop whey protein isolate – choose a berry flavor or vanilla
　　1 cup water
　　*Ice

　　For an added health boost include a scoop of wheat grass or super greens!

Instructions:

Wash and prepare fruits to add to blender. Add spinach, water and protein and blend. Add ice until the desired texture is reached. Enjoy.

Serves 2 Nutritional Value per serving: Calories: 226 g; Fat: 1.6 g (0.5 g sat fat); Cholesterol: 15 mg; Sodium: 57.2 mg; Carbohydrates: 43.6 g; Fiber: 4.9 g; Protein: 14.3 g.

Calories based on 2 equal portions of ingredients.

Spiced Apple Smoothie

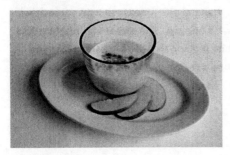

Apples are full of vitamins and minerals and drinking an apple smoothie a day could possibly "keep the doctor away!"

Add your favorite spices like nutmeg, ground ginger, allspice, cinnamon or cloves. This smoothie tastes delicious and is healthy; what a great combination!

Ingredients:

½ apple, peeled, cored and chopped
4 ounces apple juice (get a reduced sugar variety)
1 cup nonfat milk
1/4 teaspoon freshly grated nutmeg or cinnamon
1 scoop whey protein isolate – try vanilla flavor!

Instructions:

In a blender, combine the apple, milk, apple juice, protein and nutmeg. Blend until smooth. Pour into a tall glass and sprinkle a little nutmeg on top for garnish. This tasty treat should serve 2 people nicely.

Prep Time 15 minutes

Serves 2 Nutritional Value per serving: 303 calories; Fat: 1.8 g (1.0 g sat fat); Cholesterol: 35 mg; Sodium: 192 mg; Carbohydrates: 39 g; Fiber: 1.9 g; Protein: 32.6 g.

Calories based on 2 equal portions of ingredients.

Fall Pumpkin Spiced Smoothie

If you love the taste of fall, you'll love this delicious smoothie recipe.

Ingredients:

- ½ cup pumpkin puree
- ½ very ripe medium-sized banana
- ½ apple, peeled, cored and sliced
- ¾ cup "No Sugar Added" Greek yogurt
- 2 teaspoons honey – or reduce sugar by using Truvia or Stevia
- ½ teaspoon pumpkin pie spice
- ¼ teaspoon vanilla extract
- 1 cup crushed ice

Instructions:

Place all ingredients in a blender and blend until creamy. Top with pumpkin pie spice for garnish.

Serves 2 Nutritional Value per serving: Calories: 212; Fat: 1.0 g (0.5 g sat fat); Cholesterol: 15 mg; Sodium: 90 mg; Carbohydrates: 36 g; Fiber: 3.6 g; Protein: 16.5 g.

Calories based on 2 equal portions of ingredients.

A Berry Green Smoothie

Oranges, strawberries, and celery, oh my! This trio will not only be tasty, but it is also a "balanced meal" for those "on the go" mornings, or those "too busy to eat" afternoons.

Ingredients:

2 cups fresh Strawberries (frozen is also fine.)
1 orange, peeled and sliced.
1 stalk of celery
1 cup water
1 cup low sugar orange juice (or try this with water only to reduce sugars)
1 scoop Whey Protein Isolate
*Ice

Instructions:

Add all ingredients into the blender and mix until smooth. This recipe yields 2 servings. *If you want to reduce the sugar content, double the water content and eliminate the orange juice.

Serves 2 Nutritional Value per serving: Calories: 246; Fat: 1.7 g (0.5 g sat fat); Cholesterol: 30 g; Sodium: 79 mg; Carbohydrates: 33.1 g; Fiber: 5 g; Protein: 26.5 g.

Grandma's Sweet Potato Pie Smoothie

Who doesn't love sweet potatoes? Baked, roasted, and even in a pie! Treat yourself to something sweet and delicious without all the calories. This smoothie has all the nutrients and vitamins to satisfy your hunger as well as your craving for sweets.

Ingredients:

- 1 Medium Baked and Skinned Sweet Potato
- 2 cups unsweetened almond milk or fat free milk
- 2 teaspoons pure coconut extract
- 1 tablespoon Natural Creamy Peanut Butter
- ½ teaspoon Cinnamon
- Dash of sea salt
- 1 teaspoon nutmeg
- ½ teaspoon ginger
- 1 scoop Whey Protein Isolate – Try vanilla!
- 1 large cup ice

Instructions:

Add all ingredients to the blender with the exception of the ice; blend until creamy and smooth. Add ice and blend one more time. Refrigerate and serve.

Nutritional Value per serving: Calories: 310; Fat: 5.6 g (1.8 g sat fat); Cholesterol: 19.9 mg; Sodium: 282 mg; Carbohydrates: 39 g; Fiber: 3.1 g; Protein: 23.4 g.

Banana Melon Delight Smoothie

This is a great recipe for those hot summer days. It's easy to make and full of vitamins and minerals. If you don't like cantaloupe; you can substitute with honeydew or watermelon.

*Freeze banana overnight.

Ingredients:

> 1 banana, frozen
> 1/4 ripe cantaloupe or melon of choice, seeded and coarsely chopped
> 4 oz. "No Sugar Added" Greek yogurt
> 1 teaspoon honey
> ½ teaspoon vanilla extract (or try almond or coconut extract)
> 1 scoop whey protein isolate – try banana, melon or vanilla flavors

Instructions:

Remove banana from the freezer and let it sit until the skin begins to soften. Remove the skin with a knife. Dice the banana into chunks; combine in a blender or food processor with cantaloupe, yogurt, honey and vanilla. Blend until smooth.

Serves 2 Nutritional Value per serving: 200 calories; Fat: 0.8 g (0.4 g sat fat); Cholesterol: 15 mg; Carbohydrates: 31 g; Protein: 18.1 g; Fiber: 1.9 g; Sodium: 404 mg.

CHAPTER 9
SNACKS ON THE GO

*All Nutritional Values provided in these recipes may vary according to the food brand you choose and portion sizes. Please still be diligent about reading your labels and nutritional information. What it says on the label of the product you choose always trumps general guidelines!

Avo-applesauce

This snack can be pre made and refrigerated. This serves as carbohydrate and fat requirements, so be sure to eat alongside a protein source such as a shake!

Ingredients:

> Half a fresh avocado
> 1 whole apple, peeled
> 1 whole banana

Instructions:

Clean all work surfaces before starting.

Add all ingredients to either a blender or food processor, and puree.

*Tips and Suggestions: Spice this recipe up by adding cinnamon, nutmeg or allspice. This recipe should be stored in the refrigerator. Try this recipe with a variety of fruits or mix your favorites, just don't forget the avocado!

Prep time (duration): 5 minutes

Serves: 2 Nutritional Value per serving: 166.5 Calories; Fat: 7.0 g (1.1 g sat fat); Cholesterol: 0 mg; Carbohydrates: 28.6 g; Fiber: 6.8 g; Sodium: 4 mg; Protein: 1.4 g.

Calories based on 2 equal portions of ingredients.

Easy to Make Trail Mix

Trail mix is a great snack idea when portions are taken into consideration. Here is a healthy way to prepare your own at home trail mix for a mid-morning or early afternoon snack during a maintenance period. Please keep in mind that trail mix is high in carbohydrates and fat, so measure out your portion ahead of time and do not eat mindlessly!

Ingredients:

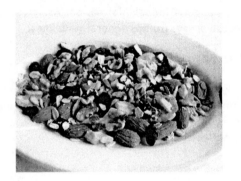

¼ cup quick cooking oats
1/2 tablespoon honey
1/4 teaspoon cinnamon
1 tablespoon sliced almonds
1 tablespoon walnuts
1 tablespoon sunflower seeds
1 tablespoon dried bananas
1 tablespoon dried cranberries
1 tablespoon raisins

Instructions:

Preheat oven to 275° F.

Mix honey and oats and form dime-sized clusters. Spread on a baking sheet and toast at 275° F for 5 minutes. Once cooled, toss in a sealable container with remaining ingredients. This is a great snack idea for the entire family.

Nutritional Value per serving: 300 calories; Fat: 9.4 g (2.4 g saturated fat); Cholesterol: 0 mg; Sodium: 17 mg; Carbohydrates: 51.5 g; Fiber: 5.9 g; Protein: 7.1 g.

Calories based on 1 1/2 Cup serving.

On the Go Chickpea Nuts

This is a tasty snack without all the calories so before you reach for that bag of potato chips, try making this simple and easy recipe!

Ingredients:

> 1 15-ounce can of chickpeas, rinsed
> 1 tablespoon extra-virgin olive oil
> 2 teaspoons ground cumin
> 1 teaspoon dried marjoram
> ¼ teaspoon ground allspice
> ¼ teaspoon salt

Instructions:

Preheat oven to 450 degrees. Blot chickpeas dry with a paper towel and mix in a bowl with oil, cumin, marjoram, allspice and salt. Spread on a rimmed baking sheet. Bake until browned and crunchy, or about 25 to 30 minutes. Let cool on the baking sheet for 15 minutes.

Nutritional Value per serving: 103 Calories; Fat: 5 g (0 g sat fat); Cholesterol: 0 mg; Carbohydrates: 14 g; Fiber: 5 g; Sodium: 303 mg; Protein: 4 g.

*Tips and Suggestions: Add these delicious chickpeas to salads or just eat plain when you are craving something. This is a great snack idea that is low in calories. You can also try smoked paprika as a spice on these. The aromatic intensity of smoked paprika would definitely add another dimension to this delicious snack. This is mainly a carb source, so would be best combined with the protein source of your choice.

Homemade Granola Bars

Why spend money at the grocery store purchasing granola bars, when you can determine what goes in and what stays out. Create a tasty and filling mini meal for you or your family. This is an item that would be eaten earlier in the day.

Ingredients:

  2 cups rolled oats
  1/2 cup agave nectar or honey
  ½ cup wheat germ
  ¾ teaspoon ground cinnamon
  1 cup Whey Protein Isolate Powder
  ¾ cup raisins or Craisins (optional)
  ¾ teaspoon sea salt
  1 egg white, beaten
  ¼ cup olive oil
  2 teaspoons vanilla extract
  1 cup of almonds
  1 cup of seedless sunflower seeds

Instructions:

Preheat the oven to 350 degrees F. Lightly spray a 9x13 inch-baking pan with olive oil spray.

In a large bowl, mix together the oats, agave nectar, wheat germ, cinnamon, protein powder, raisins and salt. Make a well in the center, and pour in the honey, egg white, olive oil, vanilla, almonds and sunflower seeds.

Mix well using your hands. Pat the mixture evenly into the prepared pan. Bake for 30 to 35 minutes until the bars begin to turn golden brown around the edges. Cool for 5 minutes, and then cut into bars while still warm. Do not allow the bars to cool completely before cutting, or they will be too hard to cut. These are also great to crumble into fruit parfaits.

Serves 12 Nutritional Value per serving: Calories: 315; Fat: 15.4 g (1.8 g sat fat); Cholesterol: 2.5 mg; Fiber: 4.3 g; Sodium: 24.3 g; Carbohydrates: 39.2 g; Protein: 9.2 g.

Calories based on 12 equal portions of ingredients.

Diana's Protein Bread

Forget packaged products like muffins and breads as they are full of preservatives and do not have the right combination of ingredients to boost your metabolism, or encourage you in your fitness goals. Diana's protein bread, a staple for such a long time on Diana's journey to fitness success, has the right combination of power ingredients, along with a truly great taste! If you are in transformation, you can make breads individually rather than in a batch (so you get the exact measurements per bread) and use the appropriate portions of foods according to the macronutrients that you need!

Ingredients:

4 Scoops Protein (try vanilla first)

3 cups Quick Cooking Oats

1 Cup Egg Whites

1 ¼ Cup Water, or ¾ cup water and 1 cup Natural Applesauce (be careful with this as there are sugars, and many applesauce varieties have added preservatives)

And here is the fun part! Depending on the stage of your maintenance program, you can choose **one cup** of the following (or mix and match for a total of 1 cup):

Cranberries, Almonds, Berries, Bananas, Walnuts.

Spice: Also add 1 – 2 tsp. of your favorite spice such as lemon peel, orange peel, cinnamon, or pumpkin pie spice, adding more flavor without adding calories.

Instructions:

Preheat the oven to 375 degrees. Lightly spray 4 mini-loaf pans with olive oil spray (or you can also use a cupcake tin to make 12 smaller portions).

Mix all the ingredients together until just blended. Bake at 375 for 25-30 minutes. Baking time can be extended or reduced depending on the consistency you would like.

Serves 4 Nutritional Value per serving: Calories: 394; Fat: 14.8 g (1.7 g sat fat); Carbohydrates: 27 g; Protein: 39.5 g. (Based on use of 1 cup of almonds, 2 tsp of cinnamon and 1 tsp of lemon peel).

CHAPTER 10
INDEX OF RECIPES

Chapter 6: Healthy Dinner Ideas

Appendix A:
Grocery Shopping 101

Tips to Know Before You Go to the Grocery Store!
1. Don't shop when you're hungry! Not only will you spend more money, you will also be more tempted to choose foods that aren't nutritious or part of your healthy eating plan!
2. Shop the perimeter. Stay mainly on the outer edge of the grocery store. You will notice that the majority of fresh fruits, vegetables, meats and dairy products will be located here. The aisles are generally filled with junk food and other unhealthy choices, which need to stay out of your cart!
3. Read, read, read! It is very important to educate yourself on what you are putting in your body. True, reading labels will take some time at first, however as your nutrition education grows, making healthy choices will become much easier. Check out the items in your kitchen before hand. Read the labels from the products that you eat often.

What to look for on the label:
*Serving Size - How much is a serving size, and how many servings are in a container;
*Note the calories, fats, proteins, carbohydrates and sugars per serving ;
*Observe total calories versus fat calories;
*Look to see what the first ingredient is on the label, this is what the majority of the product consists of;.
*Don't be fooled by confusing labels! Statements such as "Fat Free, Healthy, Carb Control, and Low Cholesterol " do not necessarily mean that a product is good for you. Read every label and don't take anything for granted!
4. Be Prepared! Take a list and have a plan! Stick to your plan, if it's not on the list don't buy it. Preparation is key when changing your eating habits and creating a healthy lifestyle for yourself. Just think how much harder it would be to avoid temptation if an unhealthy food is sitting in your home!

EATING HEALTHY ON A BUDGET

One reason we often hear for people not eating healthy is that it is expensive. But this isn't the case. In fact, filling your body with junk food, high sugar, and high fat foods increases your risk of disease. That means it also increases the number of doctor visits you have to go on, decreases your productivity at work, increases bills from health expenses and medications and so on. In fact, eating junk food in the long run is much more expensive than making healthy choices at the grocery store.

Also, some of the healthiest foods are inexpensive. When you eat smaller portions of healthier foods that actually nourish your body, you don't need to eat as large a quantity of food. You can get a large fast food meal, that is only going to keep you full for a short period of time and has no nutritional value, or you can eat a smaller, healthier meal that keeps you full for longer, helps you stay healthy, and doesn't break your bank either! What a concept!

Examples of inexpensive healthy foods:
Bin or canister of oatmeal
Eggs
Beans
Brown Rice
Frozen Vegetables
Water
Spices
Whey Protein
Tuna

Other ways to save!
Buy Generic Brands. They will cost less and are usually the same ingredients.
Buy from places like Wal-Mart/Target/Costco – these superstores will often have the same product for cheaper.
Eat smaller portions – portion control is one of the biggest reasons that we have an obesity epidemic. You cut your bill drastically by eating the amount of calories that is right for you.

ABOUT THE AUTHORS

Micah LaCerte and Diana Chaloux – LaCerte are two of the nation's top transformation trainers. Each of them possesses an endless passion for healthy living. They thrive on seeing Hitch Fit clients worldwide transform their bodies and lives by making positive eating and exercise choices on a daily basis. Micah and Diana co-founded Hitch Fit in February 2009 by launching their online personal training program which is now helping change lives in 70 countries as of the date of this publication. The duo is based in Kansas City, MO where they also operate two Hitch Fit one on one personal training facilities and have a team of 15 Hitch Fit transformers. Micah and Diana met in 2008 via the fitness industry. They were married in July 2011. In addition to being trainers, they are each WBFF professional athletes and have each won World Champion titles.

The motto of Hitch Fit is Believe – Transform – Inspire. Micah and Diana believe in helping their clients first believe in their ability to succeed, then provide them with the tools they will need to incorporate healthy lifestyle habits. Once transformation has occurred, they encourage clients to "pay it forward" by motivating, inspiring and educating the people around them to also make positive healthy lifestyle change. For more information on Hitch Fit's online training programs (which include Lose Weight / Feel Great, Bikini Model, Fitness Model, Muscle Building, Competition Prep, PLUS programs, Post Baby Programs & More) visit www.HitchFit.com. Please feel free to contact Micah at Micah@HitchFit.com or Diana at Diana.Chaloux@yahoo.com if you have questions or would like further information.

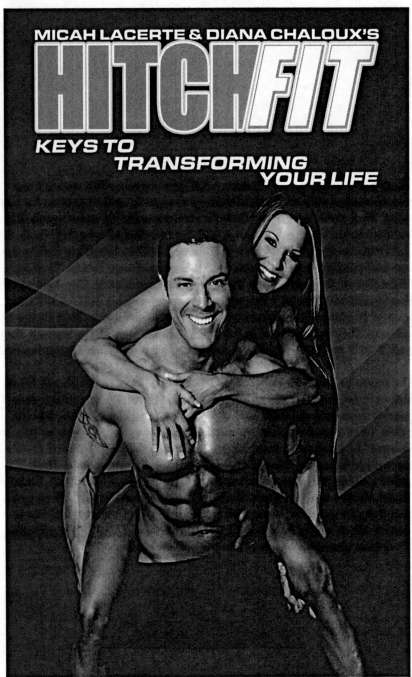

Pick up a copy of Hitch Fit: Keys to Transforming Your Life on Amazon.com today!

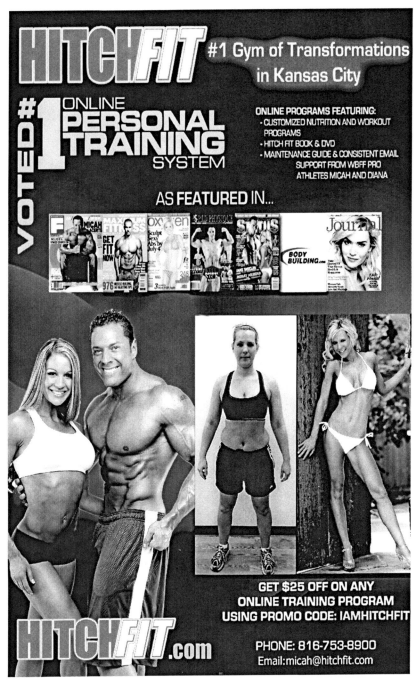

Hitch Fit - #1 Online Training Worldwide – www.HitchFit.com

CPSIA information can be obtained at www.ICGtesting.com
Printed in the USA
LVOW10s1211130714

394105LV00024B/691/P